LAP-BAND
Companion
HANDBOOK

Mark J. Watson, MD

Daniel B. Jones, MD

Distributed by: Ciné-Med, Inc.
                    127 Main Street North
                    Woodbury, CT 06798
                    (203) 263-0006

ISBN: 978-0-9749358-9-8

Notice: Our knowledge in clinical sciences is constantly changing. As new information becomes available, changes in treatment and in the use of drugs or medical devices become necessary. The authors and the publisher of this volume have taken care to make certain that the doses of drugs, uses of medical devices, and schedules of treatment are correct and compatible with the standards generally accepted at the time of publication.

LAP-BAND® Adjustable Gastric Banding System is a registered trademark of Allergan, Inc.

Printed in Canada

▼▼▼
The Authors

Mark J. Watson, MD, is Associate Professor, University of Texas Southwestern Medical Center. He is a graduate of Washington University and is a member of the Society of American Gastrointestinal Endoscopic Surgeons (SAGES), the American Society for Metabolic and Bariatric Surgery (ASMBS), and the American College of Surgeons (ACS).

Daniel B. Jones, MD, is Associate Professor, Harvard Medical School and Director of the Bariatric Program at Beth Israel Deaconess Medical Center. He is a graduate of Cornell University Medical College and is an active member of the ASMBS, SAGES, and ACS. Dr. Jones serves on the American College of Surgeons' Bariatric Network Advisory Committee, Blue Cross Blue Shield of Massachusetts Bariatric Advisory Board, and Commonwealth Expert Panel on weight loss surgery for the Betsy Lehman Center for Patient Safety and Medical Error Reduction.

▼▼▼
Dedication

The authors dedicate this book to our multidisciplinary team of health care providers who support the Weight Loss Surgery Program at University of Texas Southwestern and the Beth Israel Deaconess Medical Center. Lois Hill, David Provost, M.D., Ben Schneider, M.D., George Blackburn, M.D., Vivian Sanchez, M.D., Ed Hatchigian, M.D., Kelly Boyer, June Skoropowski, Anne McNamara, Michelle Sheppard, Maritza Avendano, Christine Lynch, Chrystyne Senkel, Dan Rooks and Ronna Casper. We also thank the nurses in our operating rooms and bariatric floor who take care of our patients during their hospitalization.

The beautiful illustrations are at the hand of Brooks Hart, many of which were borrowed from the Atlas of Minimally Invasive Surgery, 2007. We also thank Ciné-Med, Inc. and Mary Panagrosso who kept us on schedule and stewards the book to its success.

No book can be compiled without thanking our loved ones from who we take family time to write. Thank you Stephanie, Ryan, Cara, Leah, Joni, Victoria, Taylor and Olivia.

Most importantly, we thank our patients! And no doubt, with their input, we will make the second edition of this book even better. :)

Mark J. Watson, MD

Daniel B. Jones, MD

▼▼▼
Table of Contents

▼▼▼
Preface

The *LAP-BAND Companion Handbook* is a unique guide for individuals with a serious need for weight loss. As the effects of obesity on our society have become critically clear, the effectiveness of traditional diets and weight loss therapies has been shown to be less than perfect. In the last 10 to 15 years, two revolutionary surgical techniques have come together, leading the way to a new surgical option for weight loss that, generally speaking, is not only very durable and effective but also much safer.

In the late 1980s, a newer, small-incision approach to abdominal surgery called laparoscopy became commonplace. Removal of sick gallbladders, or cholecystectomy, is one of the most common procedures performed in the United States. This is now routinely done laparoscopically. Laparoscopic cholecystectomy is considered the "gold standard" therapy for this condition because it can be done with less pain and a quicker recovery, and it can decrease postoperative complications in many cases.

In the specialty of weight-loss surgery, called "*bariatrics*," procedures designed to reduce the amount of food that can be eaten comfortably at one time have been used to provide weight loss. Procedures such as the gastroplasty, also known as "stomach stapling," could initially provide some weight loss. However, the durability of these procedures was limited by stretching of the stomach and consequently, over time, loss of the restrictive effect resulting in weight "regain." At the time laparoscopy was becoming more commonplace, the second important advance, a plastic band, was being developed in Europe. When placed around the top portion of the stomach, the band, in effect, created a very small stomach pouch. When this pouch was stretched by eating, the patient was satisfied with a lesser amount of food. In addition, the band was adjustable and could be tightened or loosened as a patient's stomach changed with weight loss. The added feature of adjustability helped solve the problems encountered with stretching of the stomach and allowed sustainable weight loss.

The laparoscopic placement of an adjustable stomach-restriction band has been performed on hundreds of thousands of patients worldwide and has been shown to be very effective at long-term weight loss. The LAP-BAND® System was approved by the US Food and Drug Administration (FDA) in July of 2001. Since then, the LAP-BAND has been considered to be both relatively safe and effective as its application has grown in the United States.

Our background with laparoscopic gastric banding began in the early 1990s. We were trained under one of the pioneers in the development of minimally invasive surgery, Dr. Nathaniel Soper. When the LAP-BAND® System was released in the United States, we were trained by Dr. Paul O'Brien from Australia, who guided us as we established LAP-BAND programs in Dallas and Boston. His team at the Australian Centre for Obesity Research and Education also hosted visits to Melbourne to fine-tune expertise from their 10-year experience with the LAP-BAND®. Laparoscopic gastric banding is now a major procedure among our surgical practices.

Being faculty members at two major universities in the United States, our job is to train future surgeons in laparoscopic gastric banding and conduct ongoing research in the field. Given the recent patient demand for this type of surgery, it has become apparent that additional training is needed not only for new surgeons but also for patients undergoing placement of the LAP-BAND.

The LAP-BAND is not a quick fix. Patients must take an active role and make certain modifications to their diets and activities in order to maximize the benefits of the LAP-BAND. It is these changes that actually cause the weight loss. In the information age, the questions patients ask have often become more sophisticated and do not lend themselves to simple answers.

The development of laparoscopy and the adjustable gastric restrictive band coincided with the advancement of the Internet. The explosion of information available on the Internet is a great benefit to many. These data, however, are largely unreviewed and can give conflicting information, making interpretation difficult for potential patients. The *LAP-BAND Companion Handbook* provides a point of view not only from those in the "ivory tower" but also from those "in the trenches" in this line of work.

Today, we collaborate with the pioneers of this therapy (Jeffrey Allen, MD, Paul O'Brien, MD, David Provost, MD), develop devices with industry (Jones band introducer, closure device), and present findings to international medical societies (International Federation for the Surgery of Obesity, American Society for Metabolic and Bariatric Surgery [ASMBS]).

The focus of the *LAP-BAND Companion Handbook* is different from the authors' typical publications that appear in scientific journals and textbooks. These sources are, by their nature, difficult for the general public to interpret and contain information that might be of little interest to patients going through this process. The focus of this handbook is on the patient and what the patient needs to know. The goal is to assist individuals considering surgery or going through the process, more so than the health care provider and referring physician.

The goal for writing the *LAP-BAND Companion Handbook* was to provide a concise guide to answer the questions most commonly asked by patients. A written guide provides an instant reference for patients with questions and straightforward problems. We have attempted to avoid medical jargon and remain objective, yet share what we have learned, having cared for hundreds of patients. Information is essential for making an informed decision, and we hope to help patients embark on this journey. When the potential risks and benefits are considered, weight loss surgery will not be for everyone.

The *LAP-BAND Companion Handbook* will serve as a map and guide for those who have started, are considering, or are close to someone exploring this new method for achieving better health.

▼▼▼
Foreword

The decision to have weight loss surgery with the LAP-BAND is a deeply personal but critically important one. As in many operations, the results can be life-saving. Weight loss without surgery is an even better option but generally is not possible for people who are morbidly obese, or roughly 100 pounds overweight. This book will help you decide if the LAP-BAND is right for you or your loved one. After that, it will make the entire process, from choosing a surgeon, to the postoperative diet, to dealing with potential postoperative problems, go more smoothly. Along the way, the *LAP-BAND Companion Handbook* will answer frequently asked questions, give helpful hints, and describe potential problem areas.

I am from Kentucky, where oftentimes it seems the sun rises and shines because of college basketball. The current coach here at the University of Louisville is Rick Pitino, who also coached for the Celtics in Dr. Jones' hometown of Boston. When recruiting players, Coach Pitino says he tries to look for "basketball junkies." They may not be the best athletes or basketball players (although they are all very good), but they are lifelong students of the game—"gym rats" he calls them. These are young men who wake up and start thinking about basketball, then read a book about previous great players, go to practice, stay after for extra shooting practice, go home and watch a game or two on television, and go to bed dreaming about hitting the winning shot in a game. I encourage you to be "LAP-BAND bulldogs" before surgery. Use every available resource before surgery to know all you can about the device, the operation, and their effects.

A critical component of your research to become a LAP-BAND bulldog is this book, the *LAP-BAND Companion Handbook*. In it, Drs. Jones and Watson describe in great detail the amazing journey that you are about to undertake. Pay particular attention to the illustrations—they are well done. If something is confusing, try to visualize it with the drawings. One of the many positive aspects of the LAP-BAND® System is its simplicity compared with other weight loss surgery options; however, it is not a simple operation. The mechanics of how food travels through the pouch, Band, and rest of the stomach, as well as complications, such as a slip, are explained here with text and pictures. Many of you may remember the slogan from the old *School House Rock* cartoons: "Knowledge is Power." This book gives you knowledge, and that knowledge is the power for you to succeed.

After reading a part, or parts of, this book, you may decide that the LAP-BAND is not for you. This is okay. It is important to decide this before surgery, rather than after it. Perhaps you don't qualify for surgery for one of the reasons listed in Chapter 4, maybe coming back for frequent adjustments won't fit into your busy schedule, or possibly you just aren't ready to go on a journey as intense as this. Use this handbook to decide if the surgery is in your best interest. Only you can know that, but power your decision with knowledge.

The times after weight loss surgery are often characterized as periods of remarkable highs and seemingly intolerable lows. Complications, weight loss plateaus, and personal problems outside the realm of weight loss can frustrate patients. Buying new clothes, fitting into airline seats, increased energy and activity and even fertility, are some of the highs. Your team will be with you through these highs and lows. Refer to this book as well—it will help you through the lows and accentuate the highs.

As a surgeon, patient, supporter, advocate, and cheerleader of bariatric surgery, I can tell you that a LAP-BAND surgery is one of the most significant events in a person's life. Believe me, I see so much joy on the faces of so many patients after surgery to not give the operation and this book my ringing endorsement. I wish you the very best in your quest for a better, healthier, happier life with the LAP-BAND.

Jeff W. Allen, MD
Associate Professor of Surgery
University of Louisville

▼▼▼
Introduction

bar·i·at·rics (bār'ē-āt'rĭks) n. (used with a sing. verb):

The branch of medicine that deals with the causes, prevention, and treatment of obesity.

"Obesity is an epidemic!" You probably have seen this headline a hundred times in the last year. The numbers bear this out. There is no question that the number of obese individuals is increasing rapidly in our society. Ironically, this fact is a direct consequence of our success as a species and a civilization. We should not necessarily be ashamed of this. Our ability, as a group, to feed and care for massive numbers of people is instead a demonstration of our society's success.

For eons, we struggled as a species to gather or produce enough food to keep us alive and healthy. Looking at our collective history as a people—it is only natural to eat when food is available. Built into our genetic makeup is the experience of our predecessors that the food may not be there tomorrow, so we better eat it now. We have successfully overcome this struggle in most regions of the planet today. But, it is very easy to have too much of a good thing and overeat.

We also have the ability to recognize the negative consequences of our abundance and take action. We trace the root cause of many of our ailments to obesity, and we react accordingly. Not only is our scientific literature filled with reports on the medical effects of obesity, but it has also become a personal and popular commitment throughout our society to improve this human condition.

Obesity is a consequence of eating. Eating is second only to breathing when it comes to things that we have to do to survive. There is a built-in feedback mechanism to prevent "overbreathing"—it is called passing out. We have no way of storing oxygen for a time when there might be too little around us to use. Food, on the other hand, has an excellent storage vehicle, called *fat*. Fat is a method designed to save food for later use. Every ounce of fat stores a tremendous amount of energy. This is why it takes so long to use up the extra weight with diet and exercise. Every gram of fat stores 9 calories. Every pound of fat is about 450 grams. That is more than 4,000 calories of energy stored in each pound of fat. A hundred pounds of extra weight is almost a **half million** calories.

Since 20 minutes of running (not jogging) uses up about 250 calories, you can see how long it could take to burn off 100 pounds. Keep in mind that one candy bar is about 250 calories. Many candy bars can be consumed in the same amount of time it takes to use up one with exercise. Although exercise is extremely important, the reduction of intake is the key to weight loss.

There is now a long laundry list of conditions that can be medically linked to obesity.

Medical Conditions Associated With Obesity		
Insulin resistance Type 2 diabetes	Coronary artery disease	Cancer (breast, colon, and endometrial)
Gallbladder disease	High blood pressure	Impaired fertility
Sleep apnea	Osteoarthritis	Low back pain
Hypercholesterolemia	Urinary incontinence	Joint pain

Even more remarkable than the list itself is the experience of actual patients who have been successful in achieving significant weight loss. Many people see these conditions improved or completely eliminated with decreasing weight. Before undergoing the LAP-BAND procedure, patients may be on a number of medications, including anti-hypertensives (to treat high blood pressure), diabetes medications (high blood sugar), medications to reduce high cholesterol, anti-depressants, antacids for reflux, and analgesic/anti-inflammatory medications for joint or back pain. It is common for the number of these medications to be dramatically reduced or eliminated following weight loss after a LAP-BAND procedure. This improvement in health is mirrored by a subjective improvement in sense of well-being and self-image. Patients usually experience an increase in energy and mobility. This effect only adds to further weight loss.

Such improvements can be as subtle as allowing a patient to participate in sports or activities that were not possible at their prior weight. But they can be as dramatic as allowing a patient to have a kidney transplant or knee replacement, which they were not candidates for at their prior weight.

The knowledge that weight loss will improve health has lead to the billion-dollar industry of diet plans and exercise. Unfortunately, for many people, these approaches will not work. According to the National Institutes of Health (NIH) Consensus Development Program Statement on "Methods for Voluntary Weight Loss and Control":

- In controlled settings, diets, behavior modification, exercise, and drugs produce short-term weight losses with reasonable safety.

- Unfortunately, most people who achieve weight loss with any of these diet programs regain weight.

- Achieving and maintaining a healthy weight is a lifelong challenge [NIH Technology Assessment Conference Panel. *Ann Intern Med*. 1993;119(7 Pt 2):764-770.].

Surgical weight loss is an accepted medical option in the opinion of physicians, international medical societies, the Internal Revenue Service and the federal government. Often, the only dissenting opinion is from the medical insurance carriers who understand that obesity is an epidemic and that Americans will not tolerate higher insurance premiums to pay for it.

The following pages describe in detail surgical weight loss. Who is a candidate for it? How can you make it a part of your life or the life of someone who is close to you? As bariatric surgeons, we are on the front line of those who bring this change to people every day. It is not the intent of this book to convince someone to undergo surgery, and *this is not a substitute for a medical consultation*. The decision can be made only between you and your doctor. This book is a supplement and reference to the vast information on the topic. It will hopefully answer many questions while generating new questions that you can cover with your physician or health care provider.

▼▼▼
The LAP-BAND Candidate

The first question many people ask themselves when thinking about weight-loss surgery is, "Am I a candidate?" To answer this question, you need to first answer another question, "Am I obese?" There are as many definitions of *obese* as there are people who talk about it. In the medical field, we have established an official definition of what obesity is. It is not defined in terms of being 50, 100, or 150 pounds overweight. We define obesity in terms of body mass index, or BMI, which is a value of your weight in kilograms divided by your body surface area, estimated by your height in meters squared (kg/m^2). The NIH defines *obese* as a BMI greater than 30 kg/m^2. For a person who is 5 feet, 4 inches tall, a BMI of 30 equals about 175 pounds. For a person who is 6 feet tall, a BMI of 30 equals about 225 pounds. You can calculate your own BMI by logging on to www.asmbs.org (ASMBS Web site) and following the link, "Calculate your Body Mass Index." Enter your height and weight, and your BMI will be calculated for you.

You can also figure out your BMI with a calculator.

In the example used above, a person weighing 175 pounds, at 5 feet, 4 inches tall, would calculate his or her BMI as follows:

- Multiply the weight in pounds by 703 (conversion factor to metric units): ($175 \times 703 = \mathbf{123,025}$)
- Then multiply the height in inches by the height in inches. (This approximates body surface area): ($64 \times 64 = \mathbf{4,096}$)
- Then divide the first number by the second number: ($\mathbf{123,025 \div 4,096 = {\sim}30}$)

This gives the approximate BMI in kilograms over meters squared.

Body Mass Index	
Indicator of excess body fat	
Weight (kg/m^2)	
Overweight	≥ 25 kg/m^2
Obese	≥ 30 kg/m^2
Severe obesity	≥ 40 kg/m^2
Super obesity	≥ 50 kg/m^2

Another important measurement to factor into this assessment is waist circumference. An active weight lifter who is over 6 feet tall can commonly weigh more than 225 pounds and not be obese. The waist measurement will quickly help separate the obese from the power lifters. Simply place a tape measure around your bare abdomen just above the hipbone. With the tape parallel to the floor, relax and exhale. The tape should be snug, but not compressing the skin. Then measure your waist. This is an important measurement not only for defining obesity but also for identifying those who may be at a greater health risk. People who carry fat mainly around the waist (apple shape) are more likely to have health problems than those who carry the fat around their hips and thighs (pear shape). A person's health risk increases dramatically with a waist measurement of over 40 inches in men and over 35 inches in women. If large waist measurements are coupled with two or more of the risk factors below, the NIH recommends that something be done to achieve weight loss.

Hypertension	Physical inactivity
Smoking	Family history of premature heart disease
High cholesterol	High triglyceride levels
Diabetes	

Even if your BMI is under 35 or 40 kg/m², waist circumference can indicate a greater health risk due to high abdominal fat content.

The generally accepted guidelines for weight-reduction surgery are a BMI greater than 40 kg/m² or a BMI between 35 and 40 kg/m² with significant disease or diseases related to obesity. This translates as follows: a person who is 5 feet, 4 inches tall must weigh more than 232 pounds to have a BMI greater than 40 kg/m² or weigh more than 204 pounds to have a BMI greater than 35 kg/m²; someone who is 5 feet, 11 inches tall, must weigh at least 286 pounds to have a BMI greater than 40 kg/m² or weigh at least 250 pounds to have a BMI of 35 kg/m².

Figure A

Indications for Surgery
• BMI ≥ 40

• BMI ≥ 35 with associated high risk comorbid conditions
    - The surgeon must be experienced in bariatric surgery, and practice in a clinical setting capable of supporting all aspects of management and assessment
    - The program and patient must demonstrate a commitment to lifelong medical follow-up

Diseases of Obesity

Asthma	High cholesterol levels
Depression	Joint pain
Diabetes	Low back pain
Headache	Menstrual abnormalities
Heartburn	Sleep apnea
Heart disease	Urinary stress incontinence
High blood pressure	Varicose veins

If your BMI is less than 40 kg/m², but more than 35 kg/m², you will need to demonstrate that you have a disease related to obesity to qualify for surgery. This is known as a comorbidity. The concept of comorbidities is one that you will see over and over again in the discussion of weight-loss surgery. A comorbid condition is simply some ailment that is associated with obesity. What defines "significant" varies somewhat between insurance companies and physicians. Some of the most common comorbid conditions include high blood pressure, diabetes, and obstructive sleep apnea. Many people who are obese have one or more of these conditions that they just live with every day. They may not even recognize these as weight-related conditions. For example, many heavy people suffer from severe lower back pain, disabling joint pain, snoring, chronic heartburn, or difficulty holding their urine when they cough or sneeze. These are all significant and related to obesity. More importantly, many of these conditions can be markedly improved with weight loss. During an initial patient interview, it is unusual for a physician to not identify several such comorbid conditions.

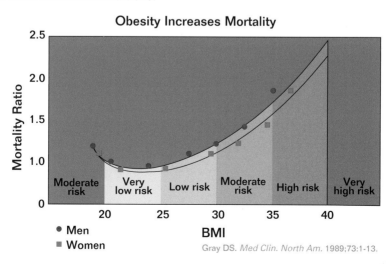

Gray DS. *Med Clin. North Am.* 1989;73:1-13.

It is also necessary to demonstrate that the weight gain is chronic. The standard guideline is that the increase in weight must have been present for greater than 5 years. Temporary or fluctuating weight is not appropriate for surgical therapy. This weight gain should not be associated with another treatable medical condition such as thyroid gland abnormality or use of medications such as steroids. We have seen patients who have had low thyroid hormone levels, and once their thyroid function was corrected, they lost so much weight that they no longer needed weight-loss surgery. Ironically, some patients become very disappointed that they no longer qualify for the LAP-BAND surgery once they lose the weight. Remember, becoming healthier is what is most important.

At the same time, your overall health cannot be so poor that having surgery would be more life-threatening than not having it done. Many times, severe medical conditions such as heart or lung disease must be treated and optimized in order to get the patient ready for surgery.

Patients Who Are *Not* Candidates for Surgery

- Unacceptable medical risks
- Untreated major depression or psychosis
- Current alcohol or drug abuse
- Inability of patient to comply with post-op medical, nutrition, and psychological management

Many patients require steroid treatment for diseases such as lupus or arthritis. It may not be appropriate for a person to have a Band placed while taking high-dose steroids. Steroids can cause problems with wound healing and infection. Chronic steroid use can cause obesity as well. Frequently, a patient's primary care doctor or rheumatologist can modify the treatment regimen in order to discontinue steroids for a period of time to allow a better healing after an operation.

Operations that you have had on your abdomen previously can also be an important factor. If you have had prior surgery or injury to your stomach or surrounding organs, it could be difficult or impossible to safely place the LAP-BAND. This has to be assessed on a case-by-case basis and may require additional tests such as x-rays or endoscopy (looking inside the stomach with a lighted scope). Sometimes this cannot be completely determined until you are in the operating room. Bands have been placed in many patients who have had prior gastroplasties (stomach stapling), which were no longer working. These repeat operations can be very satisfying when the patient begins achieving the weight loss they were looking for with surgery in the first place. Though these repeat operations are more difficult technically, the patients tend to be very motivated and understand this process firsthand. Patients should know what they are getting into and have an even better understanding of what their level of involvement needs to be in order to be successful.

An assessment of your willingness and ability to fully participate in the program is essential. If a person is not motivated to participate in the necessary diet modifications and follow-up, this can be a very difficult process. Since it is a decrease in the total amount of food that is entering your body that causes the weight loss, your cooperation is essential. The Band, the surgeon, the bariatric center, and your family and friends cannot keep food from crossing your lips. In the end, it is up to you. But you're not alone this time. The LAP-BAND will always be with you as a companion and, often times, will abate the hunger. The bottom line is that people who embrace the diet and exercise and work closely with the bariatric team tend to do well. On the other hand, the patient who is unable or unwilling to participate in the program would be better suited to another weight loss operation or none at all.

The Band will require adjustments. It makes it a lot simpler if you live close enough to your bariatric health care professional to be seen on a regular basis. This doesn't mean that you have to live next door, but if you live somewhere in Outer Mongolia, the LAP-BAND may not be a good idea for you, unless you can commit to flying back and forth. Care and maintenance of your LAP-BAND requires that you are close enough for adjustment of the Band, monitoring your weight, dealing with any problems, and assistance with your diet. That said, we have patients who live in neighboring states and abroad who follow-up with us on a regular basis and do just fine.

People with learning disabilities are probably not good candidates for the LAP-BAND unless a family member is available to assist, long term. An understanding of how the Band works and the ability to follow the eating guidelines is essential to its success. We have several patients with excellent assistance at home, and the Band works well for them.

People who are addicted to alcohol are not good candidates for the LAP-BAND. High-calorie liquids will pass right through the constriction and be absorbed. (Alcoholics typically have associated liver and stomach problems which are not compatible with the Band.) Excessive vomiting is always a real problem with Band positioning, as retching may cause the Band to slip out of place.

The original FDA approval guidelines for LAP-BAND placement in the United States required that a patient be greater than 18 years of age. Currently, Bands are being placed under research protocols in younger teenagers at some institutions. The hope is that early intervention, before chronic obesity sets in, will improve overall health in the future.

Along with diet modifications, a willingness to increase physical activity is also important with weight loss. Fortunately, patients have greater energy and ability to participate in physical activities after the LAP-BAND is in place and they have begun to lose weight. The weight is lost due to a decrease in food intake and an increase in energy expended with exercise. Exercise means sweat. Walking around the house or work would generally not constitute rigorous exercise. However, there are always exceptions. If you live or work on the ninth floor, and you don't use the elevator, that's more like exercise. Think of the whole process like an old-fashioned scale—you can choose the direction in which the scale tips.

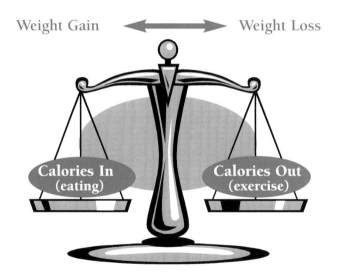

Weight Gain ⟵⟶ Weight Loss

Calories In (eating)

Calories Out (exercise)

Ultimately, a consultation with a bariatric surgeon or care provider may be the only effective way to answer the question, "Is surgery right for me?" It may require that you see other consulting physicians and undergo other tests or x-rays to get the best answer.

Some surgeons will broaden guidelines on weight requirements (when insurance company authorization is not required) to allow surgery for people who are not as heavy as the generalized NIH guidelines for candidates for weight-reduction surgery. There is currently research underway to evaluate weight-loss surgery in patients who have a BMI of between 30 and 35 kg/m^2, when severe comorbidities such as diabetes and/or hypertension are present. It may make sense to operate on people with severe weight-related illnesses before they weigh enough to meet the current weight guidelines. Improvement in the overall health and longevity of such patients may outweigh the risks of LAP-BAND surgery. In addition, the total heath care costs may be much less if the cost of expensive medications for conditions like diabetes and high blood pressure are eliminated or reduced. (It should be noted that the NIH guidelines were established before the LAP-BAND® System became an available option.)

With the knowledge of the current guidelines for weight-loss surgery and the formula for calculating BMI, you can now determine whether a visit to a local bariatric center would be a good idea for you. The nurse or bariatrician (internist) at your local bariatric center will be more than happy to sit down with you and discuss the options. Most centers have new-patient-information seminars where you and your family can learn about various weight-loss operations and have all your questions answered.

▼▼▼
A Variety of Surgical Options

In general, weight-loss surgery uses a method for either decreasing the amount of food that can be taken in at one time or decreasing the amount of food that is absorbed once it is eaten, or both. The operations are known as gastric-restrictive procedures, malabsorptive operations, or a combination of restrictive and malabsorptive.

Historically, the first such operation, performed in the 1950s, the jejunal-ileal bypass (or small bowel bypass), was strictly a malabsorptive operation. This operation worked by moving the food around the areas of the digestive tract that absorb the food so that more is passed out of the body without being used. This was simply done by disconnecting the first part of the small intestine and connecting it to the last part of the small intestine. Patients lost a great deal of weight after these bypasses. Unfortunately, patients suffered severe complications due to bacterial overgrowth in the bypassed intestine. This resulted in potential liver failure and sometimes death. Because of this, weight-loss surgery developed a bad reputation from the start.

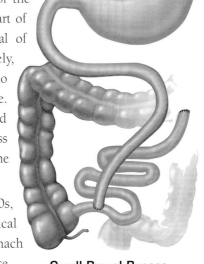

Small Bowel Bypass

Starting in the 1960s and through the 1980s, gastric-restrictive procedures such as vertical banded gastroplasty (VBG) emerged. "Stomach stapling" procedures could allow patients to lose weight by reducing the amount of food that could be eaten at one time. Because the intestines were hooked up in continuity, there was no malabsorption and patients did not die of malnutrition or liver failure. Unfortunately, the results were not durable. As the staple lines would break down, the stomach would simply regain its original size, and patients could again eat more.

Several procedures were then developed to be both malabsorptive and restrictive. The duodenal switch operations (and their cousin, biliopancreatic diversion) and the Roux-en-Y gastric bypass combine elements of both methods of surgical weight

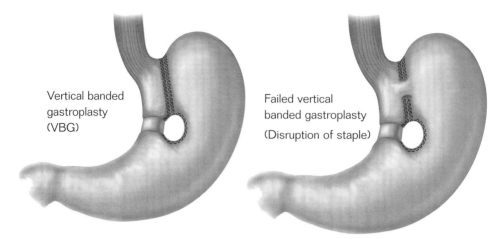

Vertical banded gastroplasty (VBG)

Failed vertical banded gastroplasty (Disruption of staple)

loss. As these procedures became more popular, the consequences of operating on very heavy people through a standard incision became evident. Immobility might lead to blood clots developing in leg veins and traveling to the lungs. Huge cuts on the abdominal walls often caused large incisional hernias. A percentage of patients also developed weight regain years after seemingly successful weight loss. Long-term, patients were at risk for vitamin deficiency, especially if they were lost to follow-up.

Rationale for Laparoscopy
Decrease pain
Improve post-op pulmonary function
Shorten recovery and return to full activity
Better cosmetic result

In the 1990s, the use of laparoscopy by general surgeons changed the face of the specialty and could be applied to weight-loss surgery. Laparoscopy is an operation done through very small, coin-sized incisions. Today, laparoscopy is the gold-standard method for common procedures like gallbladder removal. Many of the complications of weight-loss surgery were due to post-operative immobility and wound complications. Laparoscopy gives the surgeon the ability to reduce or completely eliminate such issues. The small incisions allow even the heaviest patients to get out of bed much earlier, because the incisions hurt less. For the most part, the complications associated with the large incisions in the abdominal wall were halted. When this type of surgery was applied to weight-loss procedures, the advantages were obvious. Unfortunately, some procedures done laparoscopically can be very difficult or impossible on very heavy people. There is a great deal of fat inside the abdomen that must be dealt with to safely visualize specific parts of the intestines. Fortunately, some areas inside the abdomen have less fat around them, such as the top of the stomach, where we place the Band.

Gastric Bypass

Today, the most common operations performed for weight loss are the Roux-en-Y gastric bypass and the LAP-BAND procedure. The gastric bypass involves stapling off the top part of the stomach, creating a small stomach pouch. The stomach pouch is then connected to a part of the small intestine further down the line. This operation restricts the amount of food that can be held in the stomach at one time and diverts the food around some of the intestine so that the food is not all absorbed. Connecting the stomach directly to the small intestine in this way leads to what is called a "dumping syndrome" if a patient eats the wrong foods. This is because the small intestine is not equipped to handle highly concentrated food quickly, causing the patient to feel ill. Therefore, this procedure requires less conscious cooperation to stay on schedule since the patient is punished for deviation from the menu. Importantly, nutrition must be monitored for vitamin and mineral deficiencies. It has also been observed that the intestines of patients after gastric bypasses can accommodate over time and be trained to digest most foods. Consequently, some patients, years later, regain a significant amount of weight after gastric bypass.

The LAP-BAND is very different from gastric bypass. The LAP-BAND is a type of gastric-restrictive procedure that is almost always performed laparoscopically. It is the most common procedure done internationally and the second most common procedure done in the United States for weight loss, and it is increasing in popularity. The LAP-BAND's predecessor is called the vertical banded gastroplasty. Although the vertical banded gastroplasty was effective in many cases, the restriction could be set only in the operating room. In contrast, the LAP-BAND is a plastic ring (Figure right) that contains an inflatable balloon. The balloon is attached

LAP-BAND

Stomach
Pouch

Balloon
within
Band

by a long, thin, plastic tube connected to a reservoir port, which lies beneath the skin (Figure below). Adding fluid to the port fills the balloon around the band. The enlarging balloon constricts the opening in the stomach through the band. This allows the band's tightness to be adjusted as frequently as necessary, without returning the patient to the operating room.

LAP-BAND Port

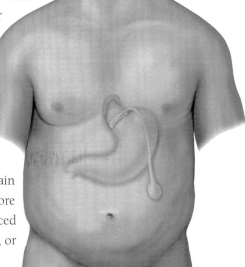

When adjusted appropriately, the LAP-BAND creates, in effect, a small stomach pouch above the Band, without dividing the stomach in half. When the pouch is filled with a small amount of solid food and distends, it stretches the stomach wall. This stretching sends a signal to your brain that you are full. Ideally, you are no longer hungry after eating a very small amount of food. As the food is dissolved and broken up, it passes through the restriction caused by the Band and is digested normally. There is no malabsorption with this procedure. Your weight loss is a result of taking in much less food than you are burning off. The chances of loss of vital nutrients are greatly reduced with an intact gastrointestinal tract.

One of the greatest advantages of the LAP-BAND is that its placement does not require dividing the stomach or intestines. This fact makes the LAP-BAND a much safer procedure than the bypass. The chances of dying from a LAP-BAND placement are less than those of dying from a gastric bypass. The LAP-BAND procedure is an easily reversible operation compared with other weight-loss procedures.

This same fact, that your intestines remain in continuity, makes the LAP-BAND more challenging to use. If you have a Band placed and decide to eat ice cream and chocolate, or worse, chocolate milk shakes all day and night, you will gain weight even after surgery. For this reason, the LAP-BAND is not for everyone. Band patients need to work with the program. If they can, the rewards are substantial weight loss and improvement in other health issues, without sacrificing normal nutrition. If you fight the Band and do not make healthy choices and lifestyle modifications, your weight-loss goals are unlikely to be realized.

BMI Chart
(pounds)

BMI	23	24	25	26	27	28	29	30	31	32	33	34	35
Height (inches)	Body Weight (pounds)												
58" (4'10")	110	115	119	124	129	134	138	143	148	153	158	162	167
60" (5')	118	123	128	133	138	143	148	153	158	163	168	174	179
62" (5'2")	126	131	136	142	147	153	158	164	169	175	180	186	191
64" (5'4")	134	140	145	151	157	163	169	174	180	186	192	197	204
66" (5'6")	142	148	155	161	167	173	179	186	192	198	204	210	216
68" (5'8")	151	158	164	171	177	184	190	197	203	210	216	223	230
70" (5'10")	132	167	174	181	188	195	202	209	216	222	229	236	243
72" (6')	169	177	184	191	199	206	213	221	228	235	242	250	258
74" (6'2")	179	186	194	202	210	218	225	233	241	249	256	264	272
76" (6'4")	189	197	205	213	221	230	238	246	254	263	271	279	287

BMI Chart
(kilograms)

BMI	23	24	25	26	27	28	29	30	31	32	33	34	35
Height cms	Body Weight (kilograms)												
147 cm (1.47 m)	50	52	54	56	59	61	63	65	67	69	72	73	76
152 cm (1.52 m)	54	56	58	60	63	65	67	69	72	74	76	79	81
157 cm (1.57 m)	57	59	62	64	67	69	72	74	77	79	82	84	87
163 cm (1.63 m)	61	64	66	68	71	74	77	79	82	84	87	89	93
168 cm (1.68 m)	64	67	70	73	76	78	81	84	87	90	93	95	98
172 cm (1.72 m)	68	72	74	78	80	83	86	89	92	95	98	101	104
178 cm (1.78 m)	73	76	79	82	85	88	92	95	98	101	104	107	110
183 cm (1.83 m)	77	80	83	87	90	93	97	100	103	107	110	113	117
188 cm (1.88 m)	81	84	88	92	95	99	102	106	109	113	116	120	123
193 cm (1.93 m)	86	89	93	97	100	104	108	112	115	119	123	127	130

Is the LAP-BAND Right for Me?

Beyond the basic questions about height, weight, and other medical problems lies the greatest question of all: "Is the LAP-BAND really right for me?"

Surgery is a big step but is only the beginning. Following this operation, your commitment to your weight loss must continue after you leave the operating room. There will be people who may be better served by a different operation or no operation at all.

> ### Why Consider Weight-Loss Surgery?
> - Currently the most effective treatment for obesity with respect to amount and duration of weight loss
> - Improvement or resolution of existing medical comorbidities
> - Prevention of future comorbidities
> - Better quality of life

If, for example, you have to have chocolate and ice cream all the time, the LAP-BAND may not work for you. This is because these foods go right through the stomach constriction and do not stretch the pouch. As a result, even though you have consumed a great deal of sugar and fat, you may not feel at all full. A malabsorptive operation, such as a gastric bypass, may be better suited for you. This doesn't mean that you can never have these foods with the LAP-BAND, but they cannot constitute a major portion of your diet.

There are people who eat continually, not because they are hungry, but because they feel the need to always eat. The LAP-BAND's most effective function is to lessen hunger. If you eat because your "very being" needs to have food continuously, this may not work for you. Even with a Band in place, you will be able to find some type of food or drink that you can continue to consume in large quantities. The only way that the LAP-BAND can cause weight loss is by making you comfortable eating less. If you choose not to eat less, you will not lose weight. Ask yourself, "If I were not hungry, would I be able to not eat?" If you think that you could decrease the amount of food you eat if you were not so hungry, the LAP-BAND will likely work well.

There are many people who are able to achieve excellent results once they have a Band in place and have the help of the bariatric team, even though they have felt addicted to food in the past. The most important factor is your commitment to making this change for yourself. Do you really want to see your health, as well as your size, change for the better? This commitment can be worth it! (See Chapter 21: *Testimonials*).

Patients cite several advantages to Band placement beyond just improved safety. The LAP-BAND is adjustable; it can be changed as you change. The Band can be removed, and you can easily be returned to nearly your preoperative anatomy in the operating room. Other operations for weight loss, resulting in re-routing the intestines, can be very difficult and more risky to reverse. The malabsorptive operations alter your ability to absorb essential nutrients. The level of these nutrients will need to be continually monitored for the rest of your life. In contrast, the LAP-BAND does not require that your intestines be re-routed, and the ability to absorb essential nutrients is preserved. If you are eating a healthy diet, vitamins are a good idea, but not essential to avoiding malabsorption, as is the case with gastric bypass.

When a person achieves weight loss with the LAP-BAND, it can be a durable solution. The adjustability can be helpful in preventing dilation of the stomach pouch, the Achilles' heel of gastroplasties. The bowel will not feel the need to adapt from being bypassed and lose its effectiveness as in Roux-en-Y gastric bypass. In general, the LAP-BAND provides an excellent maintenance program for your new and healthier weight and lifestyle once the weight is lost.

Although there are situations in which patients or their physicians feel an urgency regarding weight loss, weight-loss surgery is not an emergency. This process requires patience and planning. You will never be admitted through the emergency room for an obesity-related illness and leave the hospital having completed your weight-loss surgery. People who are very sick as a result of their weight—for example, patients who have breathing difficulties or diabetes that is not in control—need to have these acute problems taken care of prior to LAP-BAND surgery.

Preoperative Preparation
Treat comorbidities (hypertension and diabetes, etc.)
Stop smoking
Increase activity
Psychological preparation
Eating behavior
Education, education, education

A person needs to be in the best physical and mental condition possible in order to avoid preventable problems. As physicians, we must adhere to the policy of *Primum non nocere*, "First do no harm." Some patients may be too ill to undergo an operation. Turning a patient down for the LAP-BAND procedure is always difficult for both the patient and surgeon, but it may be the right decision if the patient's health is too compromised for surgery to be relatively safe.

▼▼▼
Operator's Manual

The purpose of this section is to explain, to the best of our knowledge, how the laparoscopic, adjustable, gastric-restrictive Lap-Band functions in allowing successful weight loss. The mechanics and physiology of this device will be described and diagramed. An understanding of how this tool operates will allow you to operate it safely, efficiently, and effectively for a long time.

The first and most important concept is to know where the weight loss actually comes from. Where it comes from is you. When you consume fewer energy calories (less energy) than your body requires each day, your body is forced to use up the extra weight to provide the energy it needs to function. It is just that simple.

Many people wonder, "Why then do you need to have surgery, if the weight loss is achieved only because you are eating less?" It sounds like just another diet.

The answer to this question is exactly the same as the answer to the question, "Why don't diets work?" It is nearly impossible to limit the amount of food you consume when it is working against your body's natural "set points," which tell you physiologically and subconsciously that you need to be eating more.

The LAP-BAND is simply a tool to make you more comfortable eating a shockingly small amount of food each and every day.

When you use a hammer, it is very difficult to drive the nail in if you are using the handle and not the metal head. The same is true of the LAP-BAND. If you try to use the Band to keep food out of your mouth, losing weight may be a struggle. Let's start with a short explanation of how digestion works.

Starting with the mouth, the food is broken up and moistened. When you swallow, food is pushed from your mouth into your esophagus, or food pipe. The esophagus is a muscular transportation tube that pushes the food to your stomach. Your stomach is a strong muscle and serves as a storage organ for the meal you have eaten. In the stomach, food is both physically and chemically broken up. The broken-up food then leaves the stomach and arrives in the small intestine, where bits and pieces are absorbed.

In comparison, for gastric bypass and duodenal switch operations, food from the stomach is re-routed around some of the small intestine where digestion occurs. These operations are termed malabsorptive for that reason. Some of the food that you eat (and its calories) will not be absorbed and will be passed out of your body. This causes weight loss even if you do not monitor what is going in your mouth. There are a significant percentage of patients, however, who will regain some or all of their weight after a certain period of time. If this occurs, you are now reconstructed differently and will have to monitor what you are eating.

Fortunately, the laparoscopic gastric LAP-BAND procedure is a restrictive procedure and operates on a different principle. The passage of food through your upper stomach is greatly delayed by the constriction of the Band. This distends the stomach pouch, decreasing hunger.

It is essential to understand that the restriction's primary effect is controlling hunger, *NOT* preventing food from passing through your stomach.

This is critical to understand. Patients who rely on the Band to prevent them from eating too much will many times struggle.

Eating should be approached as, "How little can I eat and stay comfortable?" *NOT*, "How much can I cram in there if I chew well?"

The LAP-BAND is a plastic (silastic) ring that surrounds the stomach just below where it joins the esophagus (food pipe). A one-ounce pouch of stomach is, in effect, created by the constriction in the stomach above the Band. The Band must be adjusted correctly for this to occur. In a way, this is a kind of stomach partitioning, without staples. The reason this procedure works, when stomach partitioning of the past didn't, is that the Band is adjustable, and staples are not adjustable. The plastic band has a balloon within it that allows the size of the opening to be controlled. The balloon in the band is connected by a long, thin, plastic tube to a reservoir outside your abdomen underneath your skin. There is a small rubber diaphragm in the top of the reservoir through which a slender needle can be passed into the interior of the reservoir. Once inside, a very small amount of sterile saline (salt water) can be injected or withdrawn. This fluid travels through the tubing and fills the balloon on the band (Figure).

LAP-BAND

Constriction can then be adjusted to a size that delays the passage of food in such a way that the small stomach pouch above the band is dilated with solid food, but the food eventually passes through and is digested normally. Dilating this small pouch of stomach causes its walls to be stretched. This stretching of the walls sends a message to your brain that you are no longer hungry. It causes a sense of what we call *satiety*, or fullness. This time, however, the sense of fullness is accomplished with a very, very small amount of food. Eating these very small amounts daily for a period of months and years causes the weight to come off, usually in a lasting fashion.

This signal resulting from the Band is actively being pursued in hopes of duplicating it with a pill, rather than surgery. Unfortunately, this new pill is not on the near horizon. At present, only surgery is likely to provide durable, reliable, and significant long-term weight loss.

The bottom line is that the patient, or "operator" of this helpful tool, will not feel so hungry following a very small meal. It is possible, however, not to use this tool correctly. For example, if the "operator" decides to consume a large quantity of high-calorie, high-fat liquids such as chocolate milk shakes, the liquid will pass right through the constriction caused by the band without providing any lasting stretch in the stomach pouch. This liquid "food" will then be absorbed normally and stored as fat on the waistline.

Another example of faulty use of this device is drinking a large amount of fluid while eating the "right" foods during meals.

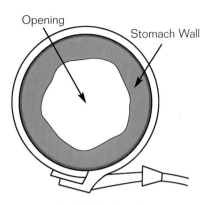

LAP-BAND deflated.
Hungry, eat large meals.

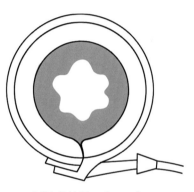

LAP-BAND adjusted.
Comfortable, eat small meals.

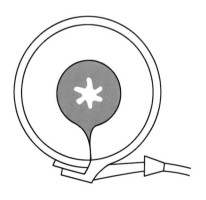

LAP-BAND too tight.
Tolerate liquids only.
Cough, heartburn, reflux.

Drinking while eating will wash the food right out of the pouch through the constriction provided by the Band. The pouch is left empty, and there is no satiety. The food will be absorbed normally and sent to the waistline. For this reason, it is always recommended that LAP-BAND patients not drink while eating. It is best to avoid drinking for an hour or more after meals as well. This allows the pouch to stay distended long enough to keep the feeling of fullness until the next meal. Keeping the feeling of satiety between meals will decrease snacking and keep the total number of calories down for the entire day. This is what causes weight loss.

Although it is important not to drink during and after meals, it is important to stay well hydrated between meals. We like to see LAP-BAND patients keep a bottle of water with them most of the time between meals. Little sips of water or flavored water throughout the day will make it less likely that you will need liquids during the meal. We also want you to stop drinking 30 minutes before the next meal to get your stomach ready.

It is a misconception that if the Band is adjusted "very tight," your weight loss will be better. We actually find the opposite to be true. If the adjustment is so tight that you are unable to keep solid food down, you will fail to lose weight and may even gain, weight, because a person will naturally gravitate toward high-calorie, high-fat liquids. Of course you can get the adjustment so tight that you can't even keep liquids down. You will lose weight in this case, but you will also find yourself in the emergency department with dehydration, and this can be life-threatening.

Situations in which the adjustment is too tight also may lead to other problems. A very tight adjustment in combination with overeating can lead to a dilation, or enlargement, of the stomach pouch and esophagus above the band. This is in effect, pulling and stretching more stomach up through the band. This enlargement of the pouch therefore requires more food to achieve the same effect. In addition, when this occurs, the opening in the stomach through the Band gets smaller because more stomach is pulled into the Band, which is a fixed ring. This makes keeping down solids even more difficult. It then becomes a vicious cycle—more constriction, more enlargement.

The most common symptoms of this pouch enlargement is esophageal reflux, or heartburn, and intolerance to solid food. More stomach acid is now above the Band, and the acid will be pushed up into the food pipe, or esophagus, because the opening through the Band is too small. Fortunately, this situation can usually be corrected (or prevented) by loosening the adjustment or removing all of the fluid from the Band and allowing the stomach to return to its original position. In some

Esophageal Dilation cases, replacement or repositioning of the Band may require surgery. If you keep your meal sizes small (1 cup), chew well, and do not have to spit up food frequently, this problem will be uncommon.

Ultimately, you are responsible for what you eat, but unlike any other type of diet, working with the LAP-BAND can be easy and comfortable for many. It can also be lasting and durable. The Band is a part of your new, healthier life. If you are struggling, the bariatric team of surgeons, nurses, dietitians, and bariatricians is available to help you maximize your results.

▼▼▼
Action Steps

Once you have determined that your BMI is high enough, and you understand what weight-loss surgery is all about, the next question you have on your mind is, **"How do I get a LAP-BAND?"** The first *Step* you need to take in order to get a LAP-BAND is to take *Action*. This is the most important step, since no one will deliver a LAP-BAND to your home. Next is *Commitment*. You have to commit in your own mind that you need to make this change in your life. You must remain committed after you have surgery and during recovery to use the Band properly. If you do not follow the lead of your bariatric center and do not follow through with the commitment, the Band is not going to function as well.

After you have committed to doing this, the next *Action Step* is to find the right team to join. You need more than just a surgeon and a plastic band. Losing weight with the LAP-BAND in place is a team effort. The members of the team include the surgeons, nurses, dietitians, bariatricians, psychologists, financial staff, and other coordinators. It is important not only to be comfortable with your surgeon but also with the rest of the team. This process is not over after you have left the operating room. You will need to be in frequent contact with the team members and involved with support groups.

To find the right team, start with the people you know. Ask yourself, "Has someone I know gone through the same thing?" A referral from a friend can be a great place to start. That person or persons could become part of your team once you have a LAP-BAND. This extended team can be extremely helpful in the day-to-day experience of having the Band. You will be able to help each other on the way to your goal. If your close friends have not been through this, they might know someone who has—ask them.

If you don't personally know someone who has gone through the procedure, there are several easy ways to find your team. There are multiple national and regional support groups that can help you. Use an Internet search with your location to find one near you. The beauty of the Internet is that even if there is no group physically near you, you can still join one. The Internet makes it easy to be in contact with others without being next door. The people in these groups may understand what you have gone through and are going through better than anyone else. They can be a great resource in finding a surgeon and center that you can work with. The

Internet will also give you access to multiple Web sites made by surgeons and centers. These can provide a great deal of information. Be wary of Web sites that look too much like advertisements for quick-fix discount centers.

The LAP-BAND manufacturer is also a great resource. In the United States, the manufacturer of the LAP-BAND® System will sell the band only to surgeons whom they have trained and observed placing bands. They know where all of the surgeons are located. Whether by phone, Internet, or mail, the manufacturer can help you find a surgeon near you (www.lap-band.com).

Don't forget your primary doctor. He or she will likely know a surgeon, or be able to find one, who can help. Your doctor can give you a referral just as he or she would for any other condition for which you need surgery. It is very important to keep your primary physician "in the loop" with this process. It is important that your doctor knows that you are making this change in your health and life. Your primary physician will need to follow you and modify your current medications and treatments as your health improves.

Another resource for finding your surgeon could be a hospital or health clinic. The hospital will know who is commonly performing these procedures and can refer you to the surgeon's office. It is important to be comfortable with the place you will be having your operation.

Recently, the American College of Surgeons (ACS) (www.facs.org) and the American Society for Metabolic and Bariatric Surgery (ASMBS) (www.asmbs.org) established an accreditation process for bariatric programs. Ask the program if they have been accredited as a Level 1 or outpatient LAP-BAND center. Accreditation requires a multidisciplinary team, appropriate resources, and a track record of good results with high volumes of patients.

Once you have found a surgeon and a center for weight control, the next *Step* is to call and make the appointment to visit the team that you might want to work with. As with many important decisions, it may be necessary to visit more than one center. The team you are calling will be committed to helping you with your weight loss. If they were not interested in helping you with your weight, they would not be offering this as a service. There are plenty of other patient problems they could care for if they didn't want to see patients that want to have a LAP-BAND. Even beyond that, the LAP-BAND procedure involves more than just placing the Band; it is caring for the person afterwards, for years, regularly. It involves Band adjustments, watching for problems, and assistance with diet and exercise activities. Even if we lose track of a patient for a while, and they return at the same weight or greater, after one or two adjustments and a little counseling, they can often be back on track. At Beth Israel Deaconess Medical Center, to encourage close follow-up, all patients sign a "patient contract" agreeing to diet, exercise, participation in support groups, and lifelong follow-up. (www.bidmc.harvard.edu/WLS)

The person you will speak with when you first call a bariatric center will know what you need to do next. They will likely want to send you a questionnaire to fill out, or they will want you to answer some questions over the telephone. It will be helpful to have some basic information ready. A more complete list of such information will be covered in the next chapter, *Homework*. Keeping your homework file up to date is a very important step.

When you arrive for your first appointment at the center, the next *Step* is to meet the team. To start with, you will likely meet a professional coordinator or nurse on the front line at the bariatric center or surgeon's office. This person will be your first contact when you have a question or need help. It is important to develop a good relationship with the coordinator and be comfortable with this person. He or she will likely be your point person. It will be a lot easier to contact this person right away if you have a question or a problem. Your surgeon is going to spend a lot of time in the operating room and may sometimes be difficult to get in touch with right away. The coordinator will know the answers to many of your questions and will know when the doctor needs to see you immediately. This person usually assists in scheduling your surgery, so it is important to befriend them right away.

Surgeon

The next member of the team is the surgeon who will be placing your LAP-BAND. Before you see your surgeon, it is a good idea to write down your questions. Surgeons, by the nature of their business, are going to seem rushed. The surgeon does understand, however, that it is very important to find out if you are a good candidate for having a LAP-BAND and if you understand what you are getting into. It makes the surgeon much more comfortable when patients have thoughtful questions. This means that you have thought about the procedure and have an understanding about the process. As a surgeon, it can be very uncomfortable when a patient has no questions. It makes us wonder if they have any idea what they are getting into. Don't be concerned if you have forgotten some questions or if you come up with new questions later. Simply write them down when you think of them and have your list available the next time you see your surgeon. The surgeon will want *all* of your questions answered prior to the operation.

It is okay to ask questions about your surgeon so that you are comfortable with him or her. It is appropriate to ask about how many LAP-BAND placements the surgeon has done. The company that sells the LAP-BAND® System will not release the device to a surgeon unless he or she has received training by a sponsored course and been observed placing several Bands. An expert in LAP-BAND surgery actually assists new band surgeons and does several operations with them in their operating rooms for their first cases. They make sure that the surgeon can do the operation safely and effectively. So even if it is one of your surgeon's very first Band placements, you could actually have one of the world's experts working with him or her in the operating room.

An equally important question is how comfortable your surgeon is with laparoscopy, or small-incision surgery. Placing a LAP-BAND is an advanced laparoscopic procedure, and the surgeon needs to be comfortable with minimally invasive surgery. Since some of the most frequently performed general surgery procedures are laparoscopic these days, many surgeons do laparoscopy on a routine basis. It also is okay to ask a surgeon the following questions:

Just ask
- How many LAP-BANDS do you place each week?
- Are you certified by the American College of Surgeons (ACS) with Fundamentals of Laparoscopic Surgery (FLS) (www.flsprogram.org)
- Did you do a Minimally Invasive Surgery or Bariatric fellowship?
- Are you a member of the American Society for Metabolic and Bariatric Surgery (www.asmbs.org) (ASMBS)?
- Are you a fellow of the ACS?
- Are you certified by the American Board of Surgery?
- Is your bariatric program accredited by the ACS or ASMBS?
- Who covers your patients when you are out of town?

It is important to know who will be adjusting your Band. This may be the surgeon who did the Band operation or another professional on the team such as a fellow, physicians assistant, nurse, or nurse practitioner. It is equally important to be comfortable with this person. They will have to use a needle for each adjustment. You need to ask where the band adjustments will be done. Sometimes x-ray or ultrasound will be required to access your port for adjustments or to check the Band itself. You should ask where you would have to go to get these imaging studies. Will Band adjustments be performed in the center's building, next door, or across town? It is a good idea to ask exactly where these procedures will be done.

It is also important to know how much the Band adjustments will cost. If insurance is reimbursing for the LAP-BAND placement procedure, will it also pay for adjustments? The center will frequently have you sign a waiver in order to make you financially responsible for the adjustments if the insurance company will not cover them. Remember to ask how much adjustments will cost up front—each could cost a few of hundred dollars. These adjustments are crucial, however, to weight loss with a LAP-BAND. Having the Band placed without care and adjustments afterwards will frequently render the whole process ineffective. Ask what the approximate average number of adjustments needed will be per year. This can vary greatly from zero to six or eight. The average for many patients tends to be around four the first year. This will vary from person to person, so make sure to ask.

Another good question is how long it takes to get in to see someone about having an adjustment or for a visit. Patients with a LAP-BAND will sometimes notice that they suddenly are eating too much and are hungry all the time. This often indicates that it is time for an adjustment, or fill. It is good if you don't have to wait a month or more to get an adjustment. Ask about the average time it takes for a patient to get in to see someone for an adjustment.

Dietitian

The dietitian is another key player of the team. If the center you are looking at doesn't have a dietitian, who will be filling this role? Sometimes it will actually be the surgeon. Frequent contact with your dietitian is necessary in order to keep you on "the program" and healthy while you are on it. How you are eating is just as critical as what you are eating, and the dietitian is going to help you. Sessions may occur during clinic visits, by phone, or in group sessions. Our dietitians find that e-mail is an invaluable tool for communicating with our patients. The dietitian will be able to help with information on supplemental vitamins and nutritional advice. They are also good at reassuring you, and your family, that you will not be starving while you are on the program. Sometimes it is alarming how little food you are taking in as you utilize your fat resources. The dietitian can make calculations and make sure that you are on course, that you will not starve, and that you will actually be getting much healthier in this process.

Financial Issues

Some members of the team at the center or office you visit will be in charge of the financial issues. Handling the information about costs, financing, insurance approval and other money issues is a complicated process. It is more than just paying for the LAP-BAND and the initial hospital and physician charges. There will be charges for office visits and Band adjustments after the original surgery charges. The cost of Band adjustments and clinic follow-up can be included as part of a yearly or monthly plan or can be paid by insurance. These are important details to cover prior to having your Band placed. It is more than a one-time charge.

For more information on cost and finance options of the LAP-BAND® System visit: http://www.lap-band.com.

An important question to ask is how additional surgery or the handling of complications will be paid for and about historical records of such costs. Though LAP-BAND surgery is safe, in general, different people respond differently to surgery, and complications can occur even in the best of situations. The financial or billing person is also going to be instrumental in the documentation process if the band placement is to be covered by insurance. This is another team player you will definitely be in contact with whether you are paying out of pocket or insurance is covering the costs.

Facility

During your first consultation, you should be able to see much of the team and facilities. You should see not only the clinic, which you will be seen in regularly, but also the facility, hospital, or outpatient center where the Band will be placed. Do the chairs and tables make you feel comfortable? Is there a dedicated bariatric clinic? Are there minimally invasive surgery operating rooms, and a floor in the hospital for patients of size? A good question to ask is, "Can the facility handle any complications that might arise during or after surgery?" "Will I need to be transferred somewhere else if there is a problem?" is another good question. "Is the ER open 24/7?" Though severe complications in LAP-BAND surgery are uncommon, it is always necessary to have this base covered. A nearby intensive care unit may save your life.

Past/Current Patients

It is also okay to ask if you can speak with current patients in the practice who have a LAP-BAND in place. The center will likely have a list of patients who would like to talk to you about their experiences. Because of the Health Insurance Portability and Accountability Act (HIPAA) in the United States, patients will need to give authorization for their names and numbers to be released to a new patient. You can get more of the inside story this way. There are also numerous Web sites that are devoted to providing information on particular surgeons and centers. An example is www.lapband.com and www.lapbandcompanion.com.

Once you have found a team that you can work with, it makes the following steps much easier. The team has been through your same situation many times and wants to help. You should be able to get your questions answered. If you are not satisfied with the answers, people, or facilities, get another opinion. It will be worth it. In larger communities, there will be a number of available teams. If that is not the case, drive to the next community to find another opinion. Web sites for LAP-BAND patients can give you personal insights into surgeons and centers.

Information on You

Not only will it be important for you to get as much information as possible during your first visit, but the surgeon/center will want to know as much about you as possible. You can greatly help your team by being prepared. The *Homework* chapter lists many of the items the bariatric practice is going to want to know about you. They will probably give you a list prior to your first visit or post the application on their Web site.

First, of course, is your height and weight. It is important to try to put aside your feelings about *the scale*. The practice has seen patients heavier than you, and they are there to help you with losing the weight. Your height and weight will be accurately measured in the center. The actual measurements may vary from your scale at home, but the office needs to have a standard reference point to make comparisons. This measurement will determine your BMI, which is important to beginning this journey.

The next *Step* will be given to you by your surgeon or bariatric center. This may include obtaining some type of test or professional consultation. Frequently, your surgeon will need some type of "medical clearance" in order to operate on you and place the LAP-BAND. This clearance might come from your regular doctor, or you may need to see a specialist, like a cardiologist. Many bariatric programs will have an internist specializing in obesity, called a bariatrician, who will evaluate your medical condition and coordinate your care with other doctors.

Part of this next step might be obtaining some type of other test or x-ray. If you have had problems or prior surgery on your stomach, you might need further testing to see if a LAP-BAND is a good idea or even possible. Ultrasound may evaluate for gallstones, stress tests may evaluate the heart, and sleep studies may evaluate for sleep apnea. These studies, when indicated, will need to be completed. This can delay the scheduling of surgery.

A screening exam by a psychologist will be required by many centers prior to proceeding. This is usually a routine part of the evaluation and has nothing to do with you in particular. Most insurance companies require psychological assessment prior to approval. In general, patients should have reasonable expectations and demonstrate an ability to commit to the program.

Sometimes the next step will require you to enroll in some type of program to document that conservative weight loss has been attempted and failed. Even though you may have tried a number of different programs, lost some weight, and then gained it back, this has to be documented. Most insurance companies will not pay until the right paperwork is filled out. This can be a very challenging and frustrating step to complete. There are some insurance carriers who will want as much as 12 months of documentation of a medically supervised weight-loss program. This can seem long but may be necessary if insurance is going to cover the procedure.

We cannot emphasize enough how important it is to join a team with whom you can follow-up. I have seen patients who have had the Band placed in another country and find their weight loss is poor until they have found a local team to join. Even if the surgeon who places the Band is excellent and cost is low, if you cannot follow-up for adjustments or other care, it may not be as successful as you would like. It may be difficult to join a team to adjust your Band and take care of you, outside of your original surgeon's practice. This is because each surgeon's team will currently be occupied caring for the patients for whom they have placed Bands. You can find bariatric centers to care for you, but it may be an out-of-pocket expense. But this expense may be necessary to get the Band to work properly and for the weight to come off.

In addition to the bariatric center, your extended team includes family, friends, and regular doctors. All should be included preoperatively, and you will need them postoperatively. You will find extended team members you don't even know yet. These are the patients in your area who have a Band in place and are part of support groups. It is a good idea, and often required, that a friend or family member accompany you to one of the new-information sessions with the surgeon.

Prospective patients are encouraged to meet postoperative patients. Ask questions! These might include:

Questions to Ask Patients

- What do you typically eat?
- How long did it take before going back to work?
- How much weight did you lose?
- Did you have any complications?
- Do the adjustments hurt?
- Would you do it again?

▼▼▼
Homework

There are some actions that you need to start right now in this effort. Having a written journal to record your personal weight history can make the whole process a lot easier. Some of the essential items to be included in your journal are discussed in this chapter.

Time Line

A history of how long you have been heavy is important. Weight-loss surgery is generally reserved for weight gain that is chronic. Chronic, in medical terms, usually means greater than 5 years in duration. This indication is to prevent surgery from being done on people who may have acute medical illness that causes weight gain. Cushing's disease and hypothyroidism are examples. Such problems can be treated medically and do not require weight-loss surgery. Weight gain with acute depression is another example of a condition that may be treated without surgery.

Weight-Loss Programs

A list of prior weight-loss programs and dates you participated in them is needed. It would also be helpful if you can remember how much weight you lost on these different programs. This log is essential, since weight-loss surgery is reserved for those who have failed to lose weight by conservative methods. It will be much easier for you to think back on all the programs you have participated in while you are at home rather than during your office visit. Old credit card receipts or canceled checks for Weight Watchers, Curves, gym memberships, or stationary bikes may help you remember.

Weight-Loss Medications

A list of any medications you have taken for weight loss is necessary. This includes both medications you got by prescription or bought over the counter. As you are probably aware, some of these medications can have serious effects on parts of your body. This list is essential not only for preparing for surgery but also for documenting your efforts to lose weight.

Medical Problems and Issues

A written list of your past and current medical problems is essential. It is much easier to list all of these things prior to visiting the weight-loss surgeon. This list is important not only to make sure that your operation is safe but also to get approval from your insurance company for placement of the LAP-BAND. Try to think of all the conditions for which you have seen a doctor in the past. Think about anything you have taken medication for, even over-the-counter drugs. Look through the list of medical conditions on page 16. Many conditions that you have suffered from may actually be related to weight.

Current Medications

A written list of current medications you are taking, including their doses, is important to keep. Any medication that you have recently stopped is also significant. Look at all the medications you have at home. Some will need to be changed or stopped prior to surgery. Some blood-thinning medications, Coumadin, for example, may have to be stopped completely prior to surgery. Others, such as aspirin and anti-inflammatory drugs (ibuprofen), may need to be stopped a couple of weeks before surgery. Steroids are best avoided during Band placement. Following your LAP-BAND surgery, your center will then keep a running tally of your medication changes. Many medications may be reduced or completely discontinued by your primary care provider as you lose weight and your health is restored.

Prior Studies, Tests

Results and even copies of previous diagnostic studies, blood tests, and x-rays are necessary. These are helpful not only for documentation but also to prevent repetition of such studies. If you carry copies of x-rays with you, this may help as well. Knowing where you have had prior x-rays is also helpful.

Surgery History

Knowing about your prior surgeries and when they happened will help the surgeon know if Band placement will technically be more difficult in you. Many prior operations such as gynecologic surgery or gallbladder removal make very little difference in placement of a Band. Some operations, like prior stomach or esophageal surgery, can make a big difference. If you have been hospitalized recently, request your discharge summary or operative notes.

Your Other Doctors, Past and Present

The names, telephone numbers, and addresses of your doctors are important. This includes not only your primary care physician but also specialists like cardiologists, gastroenterologists, and therapists. They are a part of your extended team as well. Your surgeon will want to keep in contact with them, and having their names and numbers will be essential. After surgery, they will need to adjust your medications and therapies to fit the new you, and they likely will be involved in that process.

Health Insurance Policies

Not only are health insurance cards and numbers essential but also copies of the policies. This will provide information on specific exclusions in your policy. Exclusions can make the process more challenging, but not impossible. A record of your medical charges for the current year could assist in the calculation of deductible charges. Telephone your carrier and ask if your specific policy covers weight loss surgery.

Compiling the information suggested in this chapter at the start will make this whole process much simpler. Beginning a file or journal that can be added to as you go will make this process easier and might be instrumental in the approval for insurance coverage.

▼▼▼
The Insurance Game

The next phase of the journey involves covering the cost of this life change. Patients are very interested in whether their insurance companies will pay for the surgery. The answer to this part of the question can be very complicated. There are some insurance carriers who will cover the surgery with very few questions. Other carriers categorize this surgery as an absolute exclusion. This doesn't necessarily mean that you will never get the surgery paid for by the insurance company. It will, however, be more challenging.

Before going any further, you should understand that no health insurance company will pay for a Band if the patient's weight is below the accepted standard. That standard is a BMI greater than 40 kg/m^2 or a BMI between 35 and 40 kg/m^2 with severe comorbidities (associated diseases). Band surgery in patients with BMIs lower than 35 kg/m^2 is generally paid for with cash and/or under investigational protocol.

Insurance approval is a sort of legal process. As with all legal processes, documentation is the key. The *Homework* chapter of this book is the starting point for your documentation process. Your surgeon's office or bariatric center will be intimately involved with this, but you should take an active role as well. Here are some specific things that you must do in the process of getting insurance approval when insurance providers resist.

Information must be written down to be useful in the approval process. Start a file now, outlining your current and past efforts in weight loss. Here are some things that you need to include in your file:

Copies of your **chart from your primary care physician**. There will be a wealth of information about your weight history and overall health.

Copies of your **chart from your specialty providers**. There will be documentation of your comorbidities, which can be the essence of your approval. Even if the care seems remote or unrelated, it can be critical.

Table 3. Specialties and Possible Associated Comorbidities	
Specialty	**Comorbidity**
Orthopedic surgery	Joint/back pain
Ear, nose, throat	Breathing difficulties
Gastroenterology	Heartburn
Cardiology	High blood pressure and heart failure
Obstetrics/gynecology	Menstrual irregularity and infertility
Urology	Stress incontinence
Pulmonary	Sleep apnea
Psychiatry	Depression
Dermatology	Skin rashes

Get copies of your **weight-loss clinic records or gym records**. This gives not only a history of conservative weight-loss efforts but also documentation of your weight in the past. Get all commercial weight-loss equipment and service records and receipts. This is your track record of how you have tried to lose weight and what it has cost you.

Once you have gathered all your records and history, it is time to start making new documentation. Enroll in a "medically supervised" weight-loss program. This doesn't necessarily mean seeing the doctor all the time. But it does mean that your regular doctor documents and prescribes medical, "supervised" weight loss. There are many different types of programs that will fulfill your insurance carrier's requirements.

This brings you to the next and most critical step, in which you must find out about your health insurance. You must know what is covered by your health insurance policy and, more importantly, the exclusions, or what is not covered. You can get a copy of your policy from your insurance company if you do not already have it. You can now find out what you are up against. If the wording lists weight-loss surgery as "an exclusion," the game is not necessarily over—it is just more challenging.

Your insurance is in place for your "health maintenance" or "medically indicated" services. In 1991, the NIH issued a consensus statement regarding weight-loss surgery. They endorsed weight-loss surgery for failure of less invasive methods of weight loss. The two procedures that were endorsed in 1991 were the gastric bypass and the vertical banded gastroplasty. The vertical banded gastroplasty is the predecessor of the LAP-BAND. There is currently ample evidence that the Band is a more effective procedure than the vertical banded gastroplasty, and it is considered safer than the gastric bypass.

Given that the federal government officially endorses the use of weight-loss surgery, it is a matter of demonstrating that the weight is the cause of your health problems and that diet or other conservative weight-loss programs have failed. If this can be properly presented, your insurance company is contractually required to cover the care of your health needs.

Once your surgeon has documented that you are an appropriate candidate for the Band, the center will submit a **Pre-Authorization Request** letter to your insurance company. This letter, which your surgeon's office deals with every day, asks if the insurance company will pay for having the Band placed. This is done in a routine fashion that lists all of your weight-related illnesses and your attempts to treat your weight problem conservatively.

The process of asking your insurance carrier must be handled correctly. Your surgeon's office or clinic will generally have staff that is familiar with the process. It is common for some carriers to initially refuse coverage. If this occurs, the game is not over. At that point, there is an appeal process. Your specific insurance policy will have a defined procedure for the appeal process. Many times, only three appeals are allowed; therefore, you need to use them wisely.

LAP-BAND placement has been known to be covered by the following insurance carriers. This is just a partial list. We strongly recommend that you research your own options for insurance coverage.

- Blue Cross (in some states)
- Humana
- Cigna First Health
- One Health
- Tufts Health Plan
- United Healthcare
- HealthNet
- Medica
- American Family Insurance
- Harvard Pilgrim Health Care
- Medicare

Most insurance carriers will require documentation of at least 6 to 12 months of supervised weight-loss programs. This may mean anything from Jenny Craig to your physician prescribing medications, depending on the insurance carrier.

If an appeal is filed by you or on your behalf and is denied, it is then time to get serious. The policy will grant only a limited number of appeals. In some cases, it might be worthwhile to ask for professional legal assistance. Law firms that specialize in this work exist and can help with the process, but for a fee (for example, www.obesitylaw.com).

This can be taken all the way to civil court. At that end, attorneys will tell you that in most cases, the court views insurance-covered services "broadly" (includes many things) and views insurance exclusions "narrowly" (excludes few things). Even though there is an additional expense, having an attorney may be worth it. It seems that our patients who are lawyers rarely have any problems with their own insurance approval. Go figure.

▼▼▼
Purse Strings

Band surgery is not cheap; it is still an operation that involves the operating room, a surgeon, an anesthesiologist, and a surgical team. For people who do not have health insurance, or have insurance that will not cover weight-reduction surgery even after all legal appeals, the procedure can be paid for in cash, by credit card or on payment plans.

When considering the cost of Band surgery, it is very important to consider the total costs of "the program" and not just placement of the Band. Many bariatric programs charge an up-front fee to cover preoperative education, educational materials, and services not reimbursed by insurance. Typically, the fee can range from $500 to $1,500. Other programs may waive these fees entirely. *Follow-up and maintenance of the band is critical to success.* Patients who return after not being seen for a year are often the same weight as they were the year before. After a band adjustment and some diet counseling, they get back on track and lose more in the next couple of months than they had during the whole prior year. It is very important to look at the "big picture" with this process and figure in these essential costs at the outset.

Adding or removing fluid from the band for adjustments will cost anywhere from $100 to $500 each time. Sometimes, this will require x-ray or ultrasound to locate and access the port underneath the skin. If you are going to pay for the Band out of pocket, it will be important to find out these costs before you start. The average number of adjustments will be around four the first year. Having an itemized understanding of these charges is useful. Some surgeons will not adjust a Band placed by another surgeon. This is important to know.

Visits and access to the dietitian are very important. In the end, the "what" and the "how much" that goes in your mouth determine how much weight you will lose. It will be important to know if there is an additional charge for the dietitian's services or whether they will be covered by insurance or the program fee.

For those with insurance to pay for the Band, adjustments during the "global pay period" following surgery are at no extra charge. What this means is that a surgeon's contracted fee, for a given surgery, includes all postoperative care at no extra cost to the insurance company for a given period of time following surgery. This time period is generally 90 days. Band adjustments are generally considered postoperative care by the insurance companies or Medicare and are provided free of charge during this time period.

On the other hand, if you are paying for the Band out of pocket, this "global pay period" may not apply. You will need to ask if there is a period after surgery when any additional physician's services are included in the original price. It will be very difficult for any surgeon to guarantee or warranty all such services. Individuals are so diverse that an outcome in any particular person cannot be absolutely predicted. People are not like automobiles, so it cannot be assumed that everyone will respond the same way to any particular treatment.

The patient's progress needs to be carefully followed and the condition of the Band monitored. This sometimes requires x-rays or endoscopy. The x-rays can cost several hundred dollars. This is commonly done to check the position of the Band. It is a simple and safe method for evaluating patients who are having difficulty eating or losing weight. Later on, an upper gastrointestinal series or barium swallow can make sure that the stomach pouch has not enlarged or prolapsed above the Band.

Other problems may require an upper endoscopy. This is an outpatient procedure in which your surgeon, or another doctor, looks into your stomach with a small, lighted, flexible scope. This procedure evaluates the condition of the lining of your esophagus and stomach. The cost of this procedure may or may not be covered under your insurance.

Any complications of surgery, or surgical maintenance of the band, if needed, must also be paid for. In published studies of patients with Bands, one in five will require some additional surgery for maintenance of the Band in the first 3 years. This includes minor repairs, as well as complete replacement or removal of the Band. It would be unwise to sell the farm and extend your credit all the way to get the Band placed, because there may be more expenses in the future.

The initial cost of placing the Band will vary between $20,000 and $35,000, depending on the surgeon, bariatric program, and location. It can be significantly less expensive to have the Band placed in another country, but try to keep in mind that placement of the Band is only a small part of the program for losing weight. You will need to have someone to care for you and do Band adjustments following placement. Even if you are willing to pay cash for Band adjustments, you still may have trouble finding a center willing to do them. This is not only because other offices are busy working with their own Band patients, but also because they may not wish to assume responsibility for complications, which may result from how the Band was placed originally.

There are banks, hospitals, and centers that will finance placement of the Band and allow payments over time. In addition, there are plans for maintenance and adjustments. These will include costs of the support team and professional services. Many centers will offer or can refer patients to a support center for patients having weight-loss surgery. These programs offer assistance with diet and exercise and other social support. Again, there will be an additional cost for these services. It is good to ask about this cost before you start, so that there are no surprises.

Each person and each insurance company must weigh the costs of having surgery versus the potential health benefits of losing a great deal of weight after Band surgery. Figuring the dollar amounts of operating room charges and medications that are no longer needed after surgery is straightforward. Many of the benefits of your life-change after you lose the weight are more difficult to measure in dollars.

Don't forget, many patients will elect plastic surgery after losing the weight. While some insurance companies will pay for body contouring after weight-loss surgery, most will not cover it.

▼▼▼
Getting Ready

Once the financial issues have been settled, and the bariatric office has given you a date for surgery, it will be time to get ready for the operating room. There are several action steps that you can take that can make the journey to the operating room smoother for yourself and the operating team. The area on the stomach where the Band is placed lies underneath a portion of liver. This *left lateral segment of the liver*, as we call it, must be lifted, or retracted, to show the stomach so the surgeon can place the Band. Lifting up this portion of the liver, especially in really big people, can be challenging. Because everyone is a little different on the inside, the difficulty in lifting this segment can vary from simple to nearly impossible. During laparoscopic surgery, everything is moved with long, slender instruments. Lifting something that weighs several pounds with a two-foot-long instrument that is only a quarter of an inch in diameter can be a challenge. If this liver segment were smaller, lifting it could be easier. It might not seem possible to change the size of this portion of your liver, any more than you could change the size of your foot, but that is not the case. Good data have been published that have shown that a low-calorie, low-fat diet a couple of weeks prior to surgery can shrink the size of this part of the liver. (Fris RJ. Obesity Surgery. 2004;14:1165-1170.) This can take the form of a high-protein diet supplement, of which several are available on the market. This can affect not only the size of the liver but also its "sturdiness." Instead of being boggy and easily injured, the liver can be more pliable, smaller, and less easily injured. Some bariatric programs will require you to give up sweets and junk food for 30 days to accomplish the same goals. Again, anything that makes it easier on the surgeon is better for you. It can equate to a shorter time in the operating room and less risk for intraoperative problems.

Another action that makes the procedure easier is going on a clear liquid diet at least 24 hours prior to surgery. This allows the stomach and upper intestines, especially around the areas where the surgeon will be working, to be empty of solid food prior to surgery. Some patients, especially those with diabetes, can have a large stomach, which may empty very slowly. Being on this liquid diet will give the stomach a chance to empty itself prior to surgery and reduce the risk of aspiration.

One to 7 days prior to surgery, most patients will need to have blood drawn for testing. This will depend on the type and number of other medical problems you are experiencing. Patients with significant heart, lung, or endocrine diseases (such as diabetes) may require other specific tests to look at these problems. Your surgeon or regular doctor may ask you to see another specialist, like a cardiologist, to evaluate the safety of undergoing the operation. If there is any chance that you are pregnant, tell your surgeon. Women of childbearing age can have a pregnancy test prior to surgery. More than one operation has been stopped the day of anticipated surgery because the patient was pregnant. No one wants to risk injury to an unborn child.

It is very important that your surgeon know about all the medications that you take on a routine basis. Many anti-inflammatory medications such as ibuprofen and aspirin can cause a significant amount of bleeding and should be stopped 10 days before surgery. Other blood thinning medications such as Coumadin (warfarin) may also need to be stopped and blood tests checked prior to the operation. Sometimes, a different, shorter-acting medication (enoxaparin) will need to be substituted for the Coumadin in order to protect artificial heart valves or prevent blood clots. If the surgeon and operating room team do not know about these medications, there could be a bloody surprise during surgery.

As before most types of surgery, the anesthesiologist will ask you not to eat or drink *anything* after midnight the day before surgery (when it is scheduled in the morning). An empty stomach helps prevent vomiting and aspiration during anesthesia. The exception to this rule is the need to take some of your morning medications prior to surgery. This is especially true for your routine heart medications. It is generally okay to take these medications with sips of water the morning of surgery. Ask your surgeon and/or anesthesiologist what medications you should take the morning of surgery.

Having your morning coffee, however, may get your surgery canceled. Coffee tends to cause your stomach to empty more slowly. The anesthesiologist will not want to put you to sleep with a stomach full of "latte." Some patients are surprised that not eating or drinking after midnight includes coffee. More than one operation has been canceled or delayed for this reason. For people who are having surgery later in the afternoon, it may be okay to have a light liquid breakfast the morning of surgery. Make sure you check with your surgeon and/or anesthesiologist before taking anything that morning—drinking could cancel surgery.

Many surgeons recommend that you bathe with an anti-bacterial soap prior to coming to the hospital. There are many available soaps at the supermarket. This may decrease the total number of bacteria on your skin prior to surgery. It turns out that most infections following surgery come from bacteria found on the patient's own skin. It is also important to avoid any open skin wounds, especially around your abdomen, since these will also carry higher numbers of bacteria. Shaving, for example, can be a setup for small cuts that can increase the number of bacteria. Intact and healthy skin is the best weapon against infection. Be sure to notify your surgeon if there is an open wound in the area or an infection anywhere. A good deal of plastic must be placed sterilely inside your body. We need to keep it clean and free of infection.

There will likely be another time that you will visit with your surgeon prior to the operating room. This visit can be on a date prior to surgery in the office or the morning of surgery at the surgical center. Your surgeon is going to want to answer any questions you might have and cover your informed consent.

It is important to keep an ongoing journal after each visit with your surgeon and the bariatric team. This can just be a piece of paper or the back of an envelope, but it should always be with you. Writing down any and all questions that come up during the day, or in the middle of the night, can help make the time you spend with the surgeon and other team members much more productive. Questions or concerns that seem very important at the time can completely escape you when you sit down with your surgeon or other members of the team. Keeping the journal will ensure that all your questions and concerns are covered at the time of your meetings.

There are no dumb questions! This is worth repeating. **There are no dumb questions!** No one is expected to be an expert going into this process. No question is too silly. Even a simple question lets your surgeon and team understand your concerns. There are many simple questions that have no answer at all. This is a relatively new technology and, currently, no one has all of the answers.

Your surgeon and team members will need to cover informed consent. You will be required to sign a form prior to surgery that documents your understanding of the potential risks surrounding surgery. This is not trivial, and many programs will actually ask you to take a written exam to document your understanding of the risks, potential benefits and alternatives to the LAP-BAND procedure.

The history of weight-loss surgery includes some very severe surgical complications. The LAP-BAND has been developed to reduce the potential complications of weight-loss surgery. Because your stomach and intestines are not divided during the procedure, the risks are greatly reduced, compared to gastric bypass and duodenal switch operations. As with any surgery, however, unexpected things can happen, and you need to be informed of these issues prior to consenting to surgery. Operating on people, however, is not like working on an automobile. The parts are all different sizes and in slightly different positions. The same exact operation done on a hundred different patients can give a hundred widely different results.

Following surgery, you will be on a liquid diet. Having a supply of soups and sugar-free Jell-O® for when you get home from surgery is a good idea. We are generally not concerned that you will starve while on the liquid diet right after surgery. We are also not greatly concerned about your weight loss right after surgery. The purpose of the liquid diet following surgery is to help you heal the Band in the right place for the long term. Don't spend a fortune on expensive diet drinks or protein supplements for after surgery. You will likely lose weight right after surgery and stay healthy regardless of how much you spend on diet drinks. After you have begun your solid meal program when the Band is ready, these liquid calories and protein drinks can be our albatross. They will quickly slip right through your Band and be quickly added to your waistline if you drink too many. The most important thing the month after surgery is *healing*, not weight loss.

In most cases, depending on your activity level prior to surgery, you should be able to get around okay at home following surgery. There are few direct restrictions on your activity after surgery. Many surgeons will ask you to avoid lifting more than 10 pounds or so for a couple of weeks postoperatively, but walking, climbing stairs, and getting up and down from a chair or bed should be fine. Since you will likely require some narcotic pain medications after surgery, operating automobiles or other heavy equipment is not appropriate. Trips to the store might therefore be difficult. It is a good idea to stock up on a short supply of essentials before surgery.

If you normally have some trouble taking care of yourself prior to surgery, then it would be a good idea to arrange for some help at home for a week or 2 after surgery. It is also a good idea to plan on being off from work or school following surgery. Everyone should plan at least 1 week off; you may want 2. You may need more time if your surgery requires a larger incision or if you experience a complication. Although you may be fully able to return to your regular activities in a couple of days, it is unfair to yourself to schedule anything too soon. You will have just had an operation, and it is reasonable to be sore and not want to return to work or school right away.

▼▼▼
Operating Room 101

A trip to the operating room is a necessary part of the journey of weight loss with the laparoscopic Band. The idea of having to undergo anesthesia and have surgery is unnerving for most people. We think that knowing as much as you can about the process will help ease your mind. First of all, most patients report that the pain following the procedure was not as bad as they thought it would be. Keep in mind that this is an outpatient or overnight-stay procedure in most cases. That means that very quickly, the majority of patients are comfortable enough on pain medications taken by mouth to go home.

As mentioned previously, starting at midnight the night prior to your operation, you will be asked to not eat or drink anything. This includes coffee and water. The anesthesiologist will typically cancel or delay your operation if you have your morning coffee. The only exception to this rule is that you will typically be asked to take your high blood pressure medicines with a sip of water in the morning prior to surgery. As a supplement and/or alternative to narcotics, some surgeons have had patients take 600 mg of Celebrex (celecoxib) the morning of surgery and continue for several days after surgery. In any case, most patients use very little of the narcotic pain medications.

When you first arrive at the hospital or surgery center, you will need to go over your admission information with the receptionist or nurse. It is important to know what information and documentation you will need to bring with you. This could include your insurance card or even a check. Next, a nurse will ask you a series of questions and take your vital signs. This is typically the time that you will need to remove your clothes and change into a hospital gown. In most cases, you will be asked to remove all of your jewelry, even pierced types. This is primarily for safety reasons. Electricity is commonly used during surgery, and metal objects remaining on you could cause burns. It would be best to leave jewelry at home if possible. If you have sleep apnea, bring your continuous positive airway pressure (CPAP) machine with you for after surgery.

After the nurse has checked you in the day of surgery, you will meet the anesthesiologist or nurse anesthetist. They have an important job. Not only do they need to keep you comfortable during surgery—they need to keep you healthy. If you have had a bad experience with anesthesia in the past, this is the most important person to tell. They can often modify the anesthetic to improve the experience this time. As with the surgeon, the anesthesiologist will need to explain the anesthesia and *its risks* to you. The patient must consent to anesthesia, as well as surgery. High volume bariatric centers frequently have a designated anesthesiologist with expertise in the care of patients of size.

Once you are in your gown, the nurse will probably start an intravenous catheter (IV). Sometimes a second IV is done in the operating room by the anesthesiologist. Many patients will be asked to urinate prior to going back to the operating room, or a Foley catheter, which is a tube placed in your bladder to drain urine, may be put in place in the operating room by the nurse.

At this point you will need to say good-bye to your family or friends as they see you off to your LAP-BAND journey and goal of a new, healthier and thinner life. On your way back to the operating room, the anesthesiologist may administer a medication through your IV to help you relax. Because of this medication, many patients will have no memory of the operating room at all.

MIS Operating Room

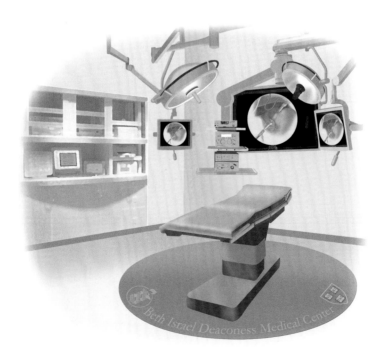

The newer operating rooms, called endosuites, are especially designed for advanced laparoscopy and minimally invasive surgery. Digital flat screens are suspended from the ceiling for ideal visualization. Voice-activated headphones control lights, the table, and the insufflator. MIS operating rooms improve visualization and make the operation easier for the surgeon. Once in the operating room, you will typically notice how cold the room feels. The nurses and anesthesiologist will keep you warm with heated blankets and other warming devices.

They will then ask you to move over from your rolling gurney to the operating room table. The operating room table will feel somewhat harder and narrower than what you came in on. The doctors and nurses will then place several monitors on you to keep track of your heart rate, blood pressure, and breathing. They will also secure several safety belts around you to keep you in place. You may feel a cold, wet grounding pad placed on your thigh. This is an electrical grounding pad for use with some of the electrical equipment. You may feel calf or foot stockings being placed, which will intermittently squeeze your feet and legs. These keep your blood moving faster to help avoid blood clots. When everything is set and ready, the anesthesiologist will place a plastic mask near your nose and mouth. It will smell slightly like plastic and is used to give you pure oxygen to breathe. You will be asked to take some deep breaths, and the anesthesiologist will start adding medicine to your IV. The anesthesiologist may ask you to count forward from 1 or backward from 100, but you likely will not make it past 5 or 95, respectively. Once you are asleep, the equipment will be set up to perform laparoscopic surgery, and the operation will start.

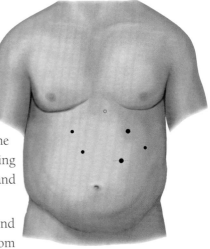

Figure 1

Incisions. A series of 4 to 6 small incisions is required.

Several small incisions will be required (Figure 1). The belly will be insufflated with air for exposure of the operative field. The Band is then brought into the abdomen as a long tube and thin strip. It is then passed around the top part of the stomach (Figure 2) and then closed by pulling the long tubing through a latch in the Band (Figure 3), much like a belt buckle.

The stomach is then sutured over the Band (Figure 4). The long tubing is withdrawn from

Figure 2

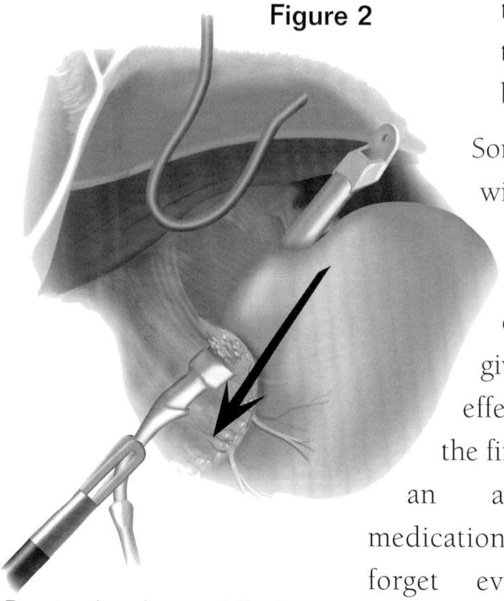

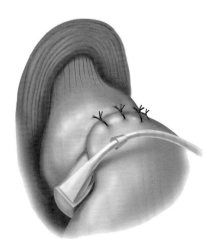

Passing band around the top part of the stomach with a laparoscopic grasper. The retractor holds up the liver.

the abdomen and attached to the port on top of the abdominal muscles but beneath the skin (Figure 5).

Some patients may be concerned that they will wake up during the operation and feel pain and remember everything. Though the newspaper press reports this occurring, it is extremely rare. You will be given a group of highly effective medications, the first of which is called an amnestic. This medication makes you forget everything. The anesthesiologist will be monitoring you closely and will be able to tell if anything is hurting you. Your vital signs, such as your heart rate, are very sensitive indicators to show if you are uncomfortable. After what will seem like a few minutes, you will wake up in the recovery room with the LAP-BAND® in place.

Figure 3

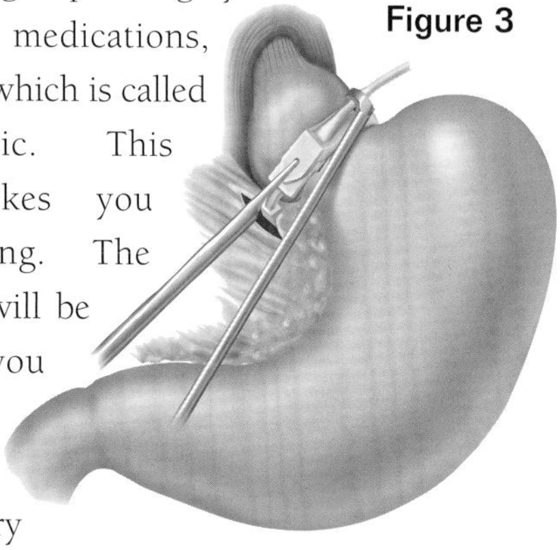

Figure 4

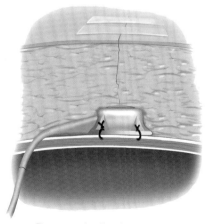

Figure 5

Port attached to band tubing

Informed Consent

You will need to sign a consent form for surgery. The process of informed consent is very important. It is the responsibility of you and your surgeon to make sure that you understand the potential outcomes and complications that can occur. All Band patients must understand that they potentially may not lose, or could even gain, weight after surgery. This is because you will be connected the way you always were. If you eat a lot of chocolate, milk shakes, or ice cream you will gain weight. Foods like these will pass right through your new stomach pouch and be absorbed as they always were.

The Band is a piece of plastic. It will require maintenance like an artificial knee or other prosthetic device. The Band does not contain any protein material, so your body cannot reject it like a transplanted organ. Everyone's body is different, however, and your body could form excessive scarring around the Band; this could cause problems like blocking off of your stomach or bowel obstructions. Ten percent of patients will require at least one additional operation in the first 3 years. While long-term data for greater than 10 years is lacking, we counsel that at least 20% of Bands may be revised, repaired, or removed over one's lifetime. Many times, however, this operation can also be done laparoscopically. The Band can develop leaks in the system that might require replacement of part or all of the Band for proper functioning. We think that complications are much less common with the FDA-approved LAP-BAND® System than with the bands available in Europe and South America in the past.

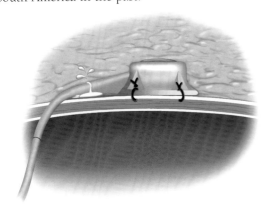

Port Leak. A needle stick can cause a small hole in neck of the port. When you go for your next adjustment you have lost your fluid as it leaked out. You are hungry. The port must be exchanged. Luckily, the Band can be left in place, so that this is outpatient surgery.

The Band can shift in its position on the stomach, causing the pouch to be too large or the stomach to block off completely. The stomach might also prolapse over the Band. This seems to occur in less than 5% of cases, but is the most frequent indication for Band revision.

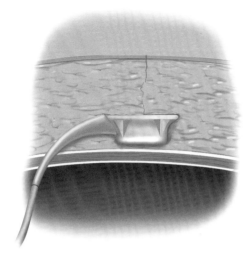

Port Flip. If a stitch breaks, the port can turn upside-down. This makes adjustment more difficult. This problem is corrected by replacing the stitch during an outpatient procedure.

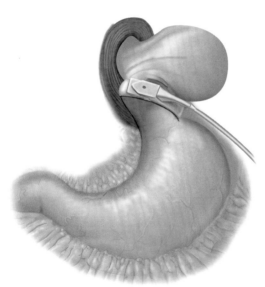

Gastric Prolapse. The stomach can slip up and block the passage of food. Vomiting may predispose to this problem. When prolapse occurs, the band needs to be repositioned or removed.

The Band might erode into the stomach. This means that the Band migrates through the stomach wall and ends up inside the stomach, rather than around it. The expected chance of this occurring is reported to be 2% of patients. We have found this risk to be much less common than this, occurring very rarely. Noticing increased hunger or a minor infection in the skin over the port are the most telling signs of this complication.

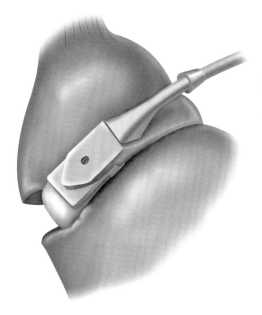

Erosion is rare, but if it occurs, the Band must be removed. Adjusting the Band slowly may prevent this problem.

Problems like Band erosion or migration are typically discovered by a contrast x-ray (upper gastrointestinal series, barium swallow) or by looking in the stomach with a small, lighted scope while you are sedated (endoscopy). If this were to occur, the Band can usually be removed laparoscopically and the stomach repaired. Replacement with a different Band could then be considered later.

The complications associated with any surgical procedure, although less common, are still possible. These would include those related to anesthesia such as heart attacks, stroke, allergic reactions to the medications, and blood clots forming in the leg veins that can break off and migrate to the lungs. Breathing problems such as pneumonia or trouble with maintaining your airway are also possible. Again, these have become rarities, rather than commonplace, but can be life-threatening.

Complications: US and International Experience Following LAGB		
Outcomes (%)	US Experience (%)	International Experience (%)
Mortality	0–.25	0–0.05
Conversion to open	0–0.2	1.3–2.7
Reoperation	4.25–10	10.5–14.9
Complications Overall Early Late	3.7–9.2 2.5–5.4 2.9–5.2	3.9–11.3 0.2–1.8 -
Perforation	0–0.5	0.1–0.5
Obstruction	1.4–4.3	-
Infection	0.6–1.1	-
Erosion	0–0.2	0.5–1.9
Prolapse	1.4–3.1	2.2–13.8
Port/tubing dysfunction	0.4–7	0.1–4.2
Explantation	0.4–0.8	-
LAGB, laparoscopic adjustable gastric banding		

Edwards M, Grinbaum R, Schneider B, Walsh A, Ellsmere J, Jones DB. Benchmarking hospital outcomes for laparoscopic adjustable gastric banding. Surgical Endoscopy, 2007.

▼▼▼
Après Surgery

Once the surgery is over, the first thing most people will remember is the recovery room. Most people will not remember the operating room at all, as you will still be partially asleep as you leave there. The first person you will likely remember seeing is the recovery room nurse. This is a specially trained person who is responsible for making sure that you stay awake and breathe well following anesthesia. The recovery room nurse will make sure you are comfortable and not sick to your stomach. Although anesthesia has come a long way, some of the medicines used could make you nauseated if you are particularly sensitive. We do not want you to vomit after surgery, especially after you have a Band in place. Excessive vomiting can lead to movement of the Band around your stomach. Fortunately, there are excellent medicines now available to help with postoperative nausea and vomiting. So even if you have had problems with nausea in the past, today you may have smoother sailing after surgery.

For people with bad sleep apnea, the recovery room nurse's job can be even more challenging, since these patients already have trouble breathing when they are asleep. Patients who use a CPAP machine at home will likely be asked to bring the equipment with them for after surgery. This may be very helpful as you awake from anesthesia to keep you breathing well. If you are spending the night, your own CPAP equipment would be best for you to use. If you do not have your own equipment, the hospital will make sure one is fitted for you by the respiratory therapist.

When you are recovered from anesthesia, you will be moved to a hospital room or to the outpatient surgery area, depending on whether or not you are spending the night. Some patients may even leave the hospital or surgery center the day of surgery and not spend the night. Of course, this depends on your age, health, who will be home with you, and how close you live to the hospital.

Allowing patients to get out of bed early is one of the huge advances in weight-loss surgery over the last 20 years. With the advent of laparoscopy, it has become more practical to have patients become mobile much earlier after surgery. We require that all patients get out of bed and walk, if possible, soon after surgery. This helps avoid a number of complications. One of the most feared in this patient group is the development of blood clots in the legs, called deep vein thrombosis. Early movement out of bed and walking causes the blood to move better in the legs and helps prevent blood clots from forming. These blood clots form more commonly in heavy patients. If these clots grow and break off from the legs, they can migrate to blood vessels in the lungs, which can be fatal. Simple activity like getting up and moving after surgery can make this complication much less likely to occur.

Developing congestion in the lungs, and potentially pneumonia, is another serious complication that was once common after weight-loss surgery. The potential of this occurring is greatly reduced by having patients out of bed after the operation. Getting out of bed prevents skin breakdown and other problems associated with immobility as well.

Your surgeon may ask that you have an x-ray before you leave the hospital. This is typically a contrast film where you will be asked to swallow a small amount of barium or other contrast liquid. This x-ray will ensure that the stomach is not entirely blocked off and that the Band is in good position. The x-ray provides a record of how the Band should look, for future reference if a problem develops.

When you are fully awake, and everything looks good, you will start your liquid diet. This could be right after surgery or the next day, depending on you and your surgeon.

As soon as the doctors and nurses are certain that you have recovered adequately to be safe at home, you will be discharged from the hospital or surgery center. It may actually be much better if you are at home than in the hospital. Being at home will force you to be up and walk more. You will also be away from the bacteria and other germs that are unique to the hospital setting.

Activity

Once you are home, again, we want you to walk and move around as much as you are comfortable with. It is okay to climb up stairs and get up and down from a chair or bed. You may be limited in what you are allowed to lift or carry for a couple of weeks after surgery. This will apply to driving as well. Ask your surgeon when he or she believes it will be safe for you to drive. Every patient may have somewhat different incisions, which affects the exact limitations. You should not drive while you are taking your prescription pain medication if it contains narcotics such as hydrocodone or propoxyphene. Of course, if you have any problems at home, you will need to contact your surgeon immediately.

Diet

When you first get home from having your Band placed, you will be on a liquid diet. This is to allow the Band to heal in the proper location. Large, solid meals right after surgery may cause the pouch to expand and push the Band down the stomach. It would then require more food to fill the pouch, and you would need to eat more to feel comfortable. In addition, the stomach inside the band will be swollen after surgery and might obstruct with solid food. This can result in vomiting, which could cause the Band to move. For several weeks to more than a month, you will need to stay on a liquid diet. When the Band is fully healed in place, then it will be safe to start your solid diet and stretch the stomach pouch above the Band. It is this temporary stretching of the stomach wall after meals that signals your brain that you are not hungry. The smaller the pouch above the Band, the less food will be needed to stretch it, and the more weight can be lost.

Having now said this, we must add that some patients will become terribly hungry in this first month while on the liquid diet. Depending on the patient's particular size and setting, the dietitian may increase the diet to include more solid foods like mashed potatoes and scrambled eggs. You should ask your dietitian before advancing your own diet. Every patient is a little different. By Week 4 to 6, it will be time to start your solid meals and get on "the program."

Incisions

Your incisions will likely be covered with an adhesive bandage or small dressing. It is important to keep your incisions dry for 24 to 48 hours after surgery, and then you can remove the outer bandage. Underneath, commonly there will be a series of thin paper strips that are glued to your skin. These help the dissolvable sutures underneath keep the skin edges together and ensure a nice scar. These strips can be rinsed in the shower but should not be soaped or scrubbed. The strips will begin to curl at the edges in a week or so. At that time they can be removed. Other methods for closure of your skin incisions include small metal staples, nylon stitches, or even clear superglue. Your surgeon will give you instructions regarding the handling of the skin closure.

After two weeks the edges of the skin are healed together. Massaging the incisions after bathing, with a good hand cream or lotion for a couple of weeks will help them heal better. Some patients have used vitamin E oil, which also appears to work well. The lotion and massage may help the healing process and make the incisions softer and feel better. Finally, avoid sunbathing and tanning for 1 year, as the ultraviolet rays will bring out the pigments of the incisions. If you are a good healer, you will likely heal well without any ointments or fanfare.

There will be a firm ridge of tissue below the skin of each incision, which may be tender, red, or lumpy. If your surgeon tells you that you have no infection, this raised area is called your healing ridge, or immature scar. Your body will automatically begin the process of remodeling these scars. This remodeling will take several months or more. Be patient as your body heals these incisions; it takes time. You also may experience some soreness in your incisions. This is especially true of the incision that has the adjustment port underneath. This is your largest incision, and the port is anchored to the muscles of your abdominal wall. You may feel some pulling on your muscles as you move. You may also feel sore next to the lower edge of your rib cage on the side of the port. Some of the incisions may appear above the lower ribs and rub over them when you breathe or move in certain ways. This should also get better as the scars mature. Anti-inflammatory medications such as Celebrex may help with this soreness and swelling. We typically request that you avoid anti-inflammatory medications such as ibuprofen in order to protect your stomach when your Band is in place.

A small amount of drainage from the incisions right after surgery is typical. Significant redness or clear or cloudy drainage from the large incision where the port is could be serious. Your surgeon or bariatric center should be notified immediately if this occurs. An infection in the adjustment port under the skin may require prompt treatment, which should not be delayed. Rarely, the port under the skin will need to be removed to heal an infection. This generally does not involve the Band around the stomach, which is in a separate location.

Medications

In most cases, you should resume your regular medications by mouth when you get home. Larger pills will need to be broken up to help them pass through the constriction in the stomach through the Band. Check with your doctor, because medications of the timed-release variety cannot be broken into pieces. You may need to be switched to a different tablet that can be broken up but should be taken more frequently following surgery. Other medications such as insulin injections may need to be significantly changed. We have had patients who no longer require insulin injections at all as the weight comes off.

There are certain things that should be watched for after surgery. Some things will require you to call your surgeon right away. A fever greater than 101° Fahrenheit may be a sign of infection or other problem. Your surgeon should be notified if this occurs. Uncontrolled vomiting after surgery is also a problem. Vomiting can cause movement of the Band on the stomach. Sometimes this can be easily taken care of by something as simple as switching pain medications. Sometimes it could be the result of postoperative swelling of the stomach where the Band was placed. This may just require time to improve but might also require that you come in for IV fluids to prevent dehydration while it resolves. Your bariatric team needs to know about vomiting.

Other symptoms should also lead you to call your doctor. Having new chest pain, shortness of breath, leg pain, or worsening abdominal pain could also be very serious. After laparoscopy, many patients will report having pain in the shoulder or shoulder blades. This is most commonly the result of the gas that is used to inflate your abdomen during surgery. The carbon dioxide gas can irritate the diaphragm, and that discomfort is referred to the shoulder area. This discomfort can be painful or just annoying. If there is any question, ask your doctor. All in all, most patients find the recovery immediately following surgery to be not all that bad. So, if you have any problems, call your surgeon immediately.

▼▼▼

"The Program"

"The program" for weight loss with the Band in place is not so much a "diet" as it is a system for eating. This can allow the gradual and durable loss of weight. It is very important to always keep in the back of your mind that the Band is *only a tool to help control hunger*. If you decide to not eat less, not to have your Band adjusted, and eat sweets all day, you will gain weight, even with the Band in place. Follow-up with your surgeon's center for adjustments and following the program is as important as having the Band placed in the first place.

At our centers, as many others do, we call it "being on the program." The entire goal of "the program" is to keep you comfortable and healthy while you consume much less food. It does not necessarily mean that you count every fat gram or calorie that enters your body. It does not always mean keeping your heart rate at 80% of maximum for 20 minutes, three times per week. It means, very simply, not drinking liquids during meals, but drinking low-calorie, low-fat liquids between meals and increasing your activity all the time. Portion control. That's it.

This is accomplished by having you eat small, solid meals three times daily. The small, solid meals fill the stomach pouch above the Band and stretch the walls of the stomach. As mentioned before, this stretch sends a signal to your brain signaling that you are no longer hungry. The pouch then needs to stay filled long enough (an hour or so) to keep the satisfied feeling until your next meal. For this reason, you must avoid drinking during meals. Stop liquids 30 minutes to 1 hour prior to meals and then an hour or more after meals. This will prevent the food within the pouch from being washed out. If the food is washed out too soon, you will be hungry again very soon.

If you do become hungry between meals, the worst thing to do is drink a milk shake. These liquids will pass right through the pouch, through the band, and into the rest of your stomach. Since you are hooked up the way you always were, you will absorb these high-calorie, high-fat liquids. The pouch will stay empty after the liquid passes through, and you will still be hungry. If you must have something, a small amount of solid food would be a much better choice.

It is important to drink lots of fluids between meals. It is hoped that these fluids will be low in calories and low in fat. For example, bottled spring water or mineral water is perfect. We like to see our Band patients carrying a bottle of water with them throughout the day. It is good to take little sips all day long. Iced tea or low-calorie flavored drinks are perfect. Carbonated drinks, however, should be avoided. These can distend the pouch, causing discomfort. These drinks also tend to be high in calories. Soda is often a large contributing factor to the person's obesity in the first place.

All Band patients will find that they have difficulty tolerating certain solid foods. Thick, heavy breads are difficult for most. Stringy, dry meats also give many patients trouble. You will have to find out for yourself what works for you. The sensations that individuals have with the Band vary a great deal. Restriction can range from a feeling of fullness in your stomach to difficulty swallowing in the throat. (Nerves in the gastrointestinal system are different from those in the skin of your fingers, for example. On your inside, sensations can refer to, or be sensed, in a different location than is being stimulated.)

When the stomach pouch above the Band is full of food, any additional food that is swallowed will back up into the esophagus (food pipe). The esophagus is not a storage organ, and it does not like to retain food. This causes the esophagus to stretch and dilate. This sensation is referred to surrounding areas. You may feel chest or back discomfort, feel pressure in your throat, or have difficulty swallowing. You could feel discomfort in your upper abdomen. Again, the feeling will vary greatly from person to person.

To make this a little more interesting, the food and amount that leads to these sensations will change as your Band is adjusted or tightened. Foods that initially went down very easily will be increasingly delayed as the Band is tightened. You will need to assess how much you can eat following an adjustment. Though it may appear that you must "give up" new foods following an adjustment, usually what you need to give up is the amount. The foods that get held up the most are the best for you to eat. They will stay the longest in your pouch, on the smallest number of calories and fat. The difficult foods can be your best friends.

As you lose weight, your clothes, shoes, and even rings will become looser because the fat gets eliminated. Similarly, your Band will loosen with weight loss This will allow foods that used to cause you trouble to slide through very easily. If this becomes noticeable, it may be time to see your bariatric surgeon to find out if you need an adjustment to tighten the Band.

If your Band is restricting you, there will quickly be a point when the next bite is too much. If you take that one bite too much, you may need to spit up the next bite. Band patients may not refer to it as vomiting, but as coughing, spitting, or burping up, often called "productive burping." This is because the food was never in your stomach. This bite was sitting in your esophagus, or food pipe. As you become accustomed to the sensation of the Band, you will be better able to judge when this point will occur. The exact sensation will be different in each person. You may need to remember how many bites you can take. Your stomach may not be able to signal you in time to stop you.

The second arm of "the program" is your activity level. Your activity after surgery is very important. Remember, natural weight loss is consuming less food than you are using up. So weight loss is equal to a combination of decreased food intake and more calories being used up. Any increase in your activity will assist in your ultimate weight loss. Start with baby steps. Don't try running for miles or swimming many laps if you are not used to it. Just walking from here to there is a start. But simply walking around work or at home does not use up a huge amount of calories. We are looking for an increase in your activity level. Many surgeons will strongly encourage an exercise target of 30 minutes daily preoperatively. This way, the behavior is already routine postoperatively.

If you have trouble walking due to knee or back pain, try paddling in the pool or exercising your arms with light weights. Any activity will help. Find an activity that you can do consistently. We are interested in the next several years, not the next few weeks. Exercise and activity level, the portion of the "scale" that uses the weight up, is the part of the program that many patients can use the most help with. While eating can be very personal and individual, exercise may work better with a group's support. Your surgeon's office or bariatric center will likely have a list of available resources. There are many commercial centers available to assist. Some centers like the YMCA or YWCA will be of minimal cost. Medically supervised exercise may also be needed as you get started.

It is extremely important to find an activity that you enjoy. If not, you won't stick with it. It doesn't necessarily need to be "fun," but you can't hate it. In that case, you won't stick with it, and sticking with it is the most important thing. You may need to continuously vary the activity to keep it interesting. Chapter 17, *Exercise and Physical Activity*, will explore this concept in greater detail.

▼▼▼
Band Adjustments

Band adjustment is critical to your program. The adjustability of the Band is what makes it unique and effective. In the past, many procedures that were not adjustable outside the operating room were not very effective. Most visits you have with your bariatric office will involve a decision as to whether an adjustment of your Band is required to improve its effect. This does not always mean tightening the Band; sometimes loosening it is best.

The decision for Band adjustment should be made with an examination of your current weight loss, eating habits, and the way you feel overall. It should not be based on a holiday or wedding coming up. It is an important health decision. Here is a partial list of factors that are used for the decision for an adjustment:

- How often are you spitting up?

  ➤ This is most critical. Further tightening of the Band in a patient who is spitting up will lead to discomfort, possible problems with the Band, stomach, or both, and ironically, weight gain.

- How is your weight loss?

  ➤ One to two pounds each week would be great.

- How hungry are you each day?

  ➤ The Band is most effective at controlling hunger. If you are not hungry, tightening the Band more may be unnecessary.

- How much can you eat at one time?

  ➤ If you are able to eat a whole plate of food without any trouble, the constriction from the Band may be too slight.

- Are you having increasing heartburn?

  ➤ This may be an indication of stomach pouch dilation above the Band. Dilation of the pouch can be caused in part by an adjustment that is too tight.

- What are your feelings and your care provider's recommendations about an adjustment?

  ➤ There is a little bit of art involved in the decision.

Once the decision has been made to adjust the Band, relax. You will feel a pinch; if needed, a local anesthetic may be used to numb the skin. After that, you will feel pressure and movement as the port is accessed with the special Huber non-coring needle (Figure D). This may feel and seem a little strange, but it is usually over quickly. Most people do not sense the tightening or loosening of the Band itself around the stomach.

Figure D

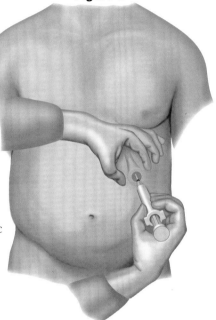

Most of the time adjustments can be done in the office. Occasionally, an x-ray machine or ultrasound will be required. As you become thinner, this process becomes much easier and faster.

As you approach the right adjustment, very small amounts of fluid are added or removed from the Band at each adjustment. The total amount that can be added to the LAP-BAND® System is 4 cc; while 10 cc can be added to the larger LAP-BAND VG. Recently, the LAP-BAND AP System™ series was released by Allergan Health in both small and large sizes. The AP Bands are slightly wider than 10 cm and VG Bands. The AP Bands have a 360-degree smooth enclosure of gastric wall by balloon to achieve essentially zero pressure at routine volumes. AP balloon fully circles stomach

An adjustment. The surgeon feels the port and can fill the port with more sterile saline (water) or remove saline if too tight.

and fills to a max. of 4.5 cc. This device is easily opened and closed for revision operations. The AP device was introduced in the United States in 2007, so it's too early to tell if it will achieve its goal of better early weight loss and induction of satiety. An adjustment of as little as 0.2 cc can make a huge difference in how a patient can eat. It is good to know how much is in your Band at any one time. However, what 1 cc is to one patient will mean something totally different to another patient. You can never judge how restricted you are based on this number compared to someone else's number. Comparing the amount in your Band to the amount in someone else's Band is totally meaningless. Everyone's stomach is a different size, and the Band comes in many sizes. Some patients need no fluid in the

Band and lose a large amount of weight. Other patients require over 3.5 cc to feel restricted.

After an adjustment, most patients need to stay on liquids for 24 hours. This will allow your stomach to accommodate to the new adjustment before you resume solids. Each adjustment needs to be lived with for a while before the decision for further tightening is made. The exception to this is if you are unable to keep anything down. In this case, you need to be seen right away to let some fluid out of the Band and to avoid dehydration and electrolyte problems.

Just as a reminder, a Band that is too tight will not necessarily make you lose more weight. If you cannot keep solid foods down, you will be forced to drink liquids, which will go right through and will not stretch the stomach pouch. You might even gain weight. Most importantly, you will not be comfortable with eating, and this will not allow durable weight loss.

> The band is not around your lips, it is around your stomach. It cannot keep food out of your mouth. Only you can do that.

You may or may not be able to feel your adjustment port under the skin. (Some patients do not ever feel the port.) For some patients, the location can be irritating if it is close to the belt or bra line. Occasionally, we need to move the port location for these reasons. This is typically an outpatient procedure. Some patients will lose so much weight that the port sticks out and becomes noticeable and uncomfortable. Again, the port can be changed to a low-profile model as an outpatient procedure. Immediately after surgery, the healing ridge mentioned earlier may obscure the opening for the adjustment needle. In this case, your doctor will need to use an x-ray or ultrasound machine to locate and access the port. After the scar has matured and you are thinner, this will not be necessary. Occasionally, the tubing coming out of the port can become kinked or broken. The port could flip over or not be accessible for other reasons. Although these problems are uncommon, the port may have to be changed for any of these reasons as well. The adjustment port must be in good position and functioning.

Try not to fear Band adjustments. Having someone come at you with a needle will never be inviting, but it will become easier with each adjustment. Remember that each adjustment is bringing you one step closer to achieving your goal—your new health and body.

Stay the Course

It is much easier said than done, but patience is very important in weight loss with the Band. Although it may seem like weight was added overnight, it took time to gain the weight. It takes time to lose the weight as well. The Band allows you to lose weight by helping you decrease your intake. That is all it can do. The rest is up to you. If you are able to follow the program and increase your daily physical activity, you could see a one- to two- pound weight loss each week. Some weeks will show more weight loss, some less. It is important to keep in view a reasonable target weight over a reasonable time period. The dietitian will help you. You can succeed!

Statistically, it is reasonable to expect a 40% to 50% loss of excess body weight in the first 2 years with the Band. This is not the ceiling, this is the average seen over large numbers of patients. You could see more, and it is possible to have less. The Band is a tool, and its results depend on how you use it. Say your height is 5 feet, 5 inches, and your starting weight was 290 pounds. By the charts, your ideal body weight will be 150 pounds. This gives you an excess body weight of 140 pounds. It is reasonable to expect a loss of half this excess weight during the first 2 years. That means that we would like to see you at about 220 pounds after 2 years, by losing one half of excess weight, or 70 pounds. But this will require healthy food choices, small portions, and exercise.

EWL: US and International Experience Following LAGB		
Outcomes (%)	US Experience (%)	International Experience (%)
EWL (years) 1 2 3 4-5	41-48 46-52 53-62 64	37-52 52 55 52-74
EWL, excess weight loss; **LAGB,** laparoscopic adjustable gastric banding		

Edwards M, Grinbaum R, Schneider B, Walsh A, Ellsmere J, Jones DB. Benchmarking hospital outcomes for laparoscopic adjustable gastric banding. Surgical Endoscopy, 2007.

This is not the most you can lose, but rather a reasonable goal at 2 years. The beauty of the Band is that patients can continue to lose weight after this first benchmark is reached. Many other weight-loss surgeries see weight regain after this point. The international groups have shown a linear weight loss over ten years. It is really up to you. The Band will make it comfortable to measurably decrease your food intake. As your weight decreases, you will have more energy and be better able to participate in greater physical activities. The increased activity is important to ongoing weight loss.

Even more dramatic than the number of pounds lost is the improvement you will see in your health. If you started out on medications for high blood pressure and diabetes, often you will see the need for these medicines reduced or completely eliminated. Just imagine not needing that pile of pills every morning. We see this frequently following Band placement. Many people who required insulin injections for adult-onset diabetes will no longer require shots. Patients with sleep apnea, who required machines at night to help them breathe throw away the CPAP machines. People who were unable to walk due to knees and hips that would not carry their weight start to jog. The following table illustrates the most recent cohort study at 2 years at Beth Israel Deaconess Medical Center.

Resolution of obesity-related comorbidities with weight loss 2 years following LAP-BAND			
Comorbidity	Resolved	Improved	Unchanged
Diabetes	74%	16%	10%
Hypertension	57%	25%	18%
GERD	55%	18%	27%
Dyslipidemia	38%	38%	24%
GERD, gastroesophageal reflux disease			

Edwards M, Grinbaum R, Schneider B, Walsh A, Ellsmere J, Jones DB. Benchmarking hospital outcomes for laparoscopic adjustable gastric banding. Surgical Endoscopy, 2007.

To reach the new state of improved quality of health requires your cooperation. Keeping your follow-up appointments with your team is critical. Even if you do not need a Band adjustment, your surgeon or dietitian can usually find simple ways to increase your weight loss. By making small changes in the way you're eating, not necessarily what you're eating, you can improve the process. Commonly, we find that patients whose weight loss has slowed only need to change the way they are drinking liquids during the day or decrease the number of times they have meals during the day to reduce the total amount of food taken in daily.

Occasionally, patients will become frustrated a year after their Bands were placed when their weight loss slows. When we sit down and look at their weight loss, we frequently find that they have statistically achieved a reasonable 2-year goal in 1 year. They are ahead of schedule, and this explains why their weight loss has slowed. Further weight loss is then possible by staying the course and being patient.

At any time in this process, increasing weight loss is possible in two ways:

- Increasing daily activity and burning more calories
- Decreasing the total number of daily calories consumed

A small change in both at the same time will be the most effective. Walking one extra block and changing between-meal liquids to ones without calories, like water, will make the difference. You will notice no change overnight. This has to be a daily change. Small steps at a time. Many patients will take a "before" and "after" photo. Over time, as you stay the course, it can be very rewarding to track your progress.

▼▼▼
Eating Healthy After the LAP-BAND

As you choose a healthy diet and eat smaller portions, your energy (caloric) intake will be less. Utilizing energy by exercising will further consume energy and burn fat stores (See Chapter 17, *Exercise and Physical Activity*). The wonderful thing about the Band is that it does not require going on a traditional diet, and you need not go crazy counting calories or fat grams with every bite. But you do need to avoid "junk" food, sweets, and chocolate and make HEALTHY food choices as part of a healthy lifestyle. Dietitians are essential to a comprehensive bariatric program, your nutritional education, and ultimately your successful weight loss.

Physiologically, unlike the gastric bypass operation for weight loss, after the LAP-BAND your intestines remain in continuity, and you do not have to worry about side effects of dumping. However, you may still vomit or regurgitate if you eat too much too fast. Breads, rice, pasta, stringy vegetables, and tough, dry meats may still be difficult to eat.

Most patients can make diet modifications. Developing the habit of eating slowly and, very small amounts of the healthy foods you enjoy is the key. There are different phases to the LAP-BAND diet, with different purposes. Understanding the purposes of the phases is critical.

Phase One: Right After Surgery

Immediately after your LAP-BAND is placed, you will start on a liquid diet. We want to get you to rethink your relationship with food. The main purpose of this diet is not punishment, but we want the LAP-BAND to heal in position where it was placed in the operating room. Consuming solid food right after surgery might cause the Band to shift its position on the stomach. Solid food might also make you regurgitate which also could cause the Band to slip.

Because the purpose of the liquid diet is to heal the Band in place, weight loss during postoperative recuperation may occur, but it is not the primary goal. You will have the Band for years, and having it in good position is most critical. Most patients will indeed lose weight, but that is not the primary goal in the first month.

Some patients will leave the hospital on what we term as a "full liquid diet." This diet will include more variety than just gelatin, and includes low fat liquid dairy products, strained low fat soups, and protein supplements. We advise that you taste test these foods and supplements prior to surgery but not spend a huge amount of money on protein supplements for the period of time right after surgery. Liquid foods and supplements should be limited once you are on a solid diet program. This is because these foods will go right through the constriction in the Band and liquids will not fill you up.

Here is an incomplete list of items that may be included in a "full liquid diet." You must check with your bariatric center for the complete list and suggestions. This list may vary for individual patients.

- Water
- Low fat liquid dairy products
- Low sugar protein supplements
- Decaffeinated tea
- Bouillon or broth
- Strained low fat cream soup
- Low fat, low sugar pudding
- Diet gelatin
- Low sugar frozen pop

Phase Two: the Soft Diet

Several weeks after surgery (this might vary between centers) you may be advanced to a soft diet. This will be most welcomed by many Band patients who feel that they may be "starving" drinking only liquids. The thicker the consistency of the food, the greater filling and sense of fullness in the stomach pouch above the Band. Foods included in the soft diet include:

Foods on the full liquid diet plus:

- Thin scrambled eggs
- Thin mashed potatoes, no skins
- Well-cooked vegetables without skin
- Soft, ripened fruits (applesauce, canned pears)
- Hot cereals (cream of wheat, oatmeal)
- Low fat cottage cheese/yogurt

The Final Phase: Regular Food

On the final diet, the key is to feel satisfied following a very small (2–4 ounce) amount of food while meeting protein goals (60–80 grams daily). Another important element of this plan is to avoid drinking liquids during, or 30 to 60 minutes after, meals. This prevents the food you have eaten from being washed out of the pouch above the Band.

We will refer to meal sizes in terms of numbers or fractions of cups, or ounces (1 cup = 8 ounces). Each ounce equates to about two tablespoons. It is important to keep in mind that many people's typical "bite" may be bigger than one tablespoon, therefore, understanding portion size is a must. Using measuring cups and spoons will be invaluable tools to better estimate portions. Also, the firmer the consistency of the food, the better your sense of fullness will be after eating and the longer you are likely to be satisfied prior to your next meal. Protein should be a priority at meal time to also help you feel full.

While many patients eat for reasons other than hunger, the goal of the LAP-BAND is to achieve satiety and restriction without vomiting or regurgitation. The first meal in the morning may be a challenge for many, but as the day goes on, eating is easier. The reasons are not entirely clear, but some modification of the diet will many times be necessary.

Sometimes, beginning with a warm liquid like decaffeinated tea might loosen things up. Several tablespoons of hot cereal or low fat yogurt may also be a good start. Firmer foods may be difficult. If the choice is something soft or nothing at all, it is better for you to eat something, so that you are not overly hungry before lunch. If you are able to eat in the morning without trouble, start with a scrambled or poached egg and a half a piece of whole wheat toast or a small portion of lox with low fat cream cheese. When you are eating a small portion of healthy foods and exercising regularly, you do not need to count calories or fat grams to help you lose weight.

An hour after breakfast and until 30 minutes before lunch is the time to focus on drinking plenty of fluids. Having a bottle of decaffeinated, sugar-free, non-carbonated fluid with you at all times is a good idea. Juices, sweetened drinks, or soda can sneak literally hundreds of calories into your day that you might not notice. Eight cups of fluid a day is a good guideline for healthy fluid intake. As your body is being remodeled, waste products are produced, which must be eliminated. Much of this elimination will be done through the kidneys, which require water for the process to work efficiently. Keep the bottle with you as much as possible.

If you become too hungry between meals, you may need to have a snack.

Snacking is discouraged, but it might help you from eating too much at the next meal. It is essential to choose snacks that don't contain a bunch of "empty calories," such as chocolate, ice cream, chips, and cheese puffs. This is another situation where the Band can be defeated. You can eat three of the smallest, healthiest meals during the day, but you can easily counteract your efforts with consuming high calorie food between meals. Therefore, it is essential to keep tabs on your snacks.

The ideal snacks are low in calories and saturated fat, such as, 1/2 peeled apple with 1 ounce low fat cheese or low fat cottage cheese and 1/2 cup berries or peaches. Vegetable sticks may be too stringy to be comfortably digested.

The mid-day meal is critical. This is because many people have skimped on breakfast and are now overly hungry. Many people will also be at work or out for this meal, and food choices may be more difficult. If you keep the mantra however;

- small,

- solid meals,

- no drinking,

- proteins first,

you should be okay.

Think about your measuring cup (8 ounces) and two tablespoons per ounce. Start filling your cup with protein first. The best choices (e.g., baked chicken or fish with cooked tender vegetables and soft fruits) may be hardest for you to comfortably digest. Many Band patients have difficulty with foods that are tough and dry (i.e., meat) as well as rice, pasta, bread, and stringy vegetables. Therefore, choose small portions of moist and tender solid foods; chew your foods thoroughly, and take at least 20 to 30 minutes to eat your meal. If you take less than 20 minutes to eat your food, your stomach may not be able to signal your brain that you are full and then you may overeat. You need to remember to listen to your body or sense of fullness, as your last bite can be too much.

Two to three ounces of the meat with 1/2 cup cooked vegetables should be fine. For vegetarians, a couple of ounces of tofu or a scrambled egg may work. Remember not to drink while eating and try to wait an hour after a meal before drinking.

The goal at the evening meal will be the same. Remember the mantra:

- small,
- solid meals,
- no drinking,
- proteins first,

you should be okay.

Salads are a healthy choice; add a few slices of grilled chicken or other protein foods to help keep yourself full. Since salads are mostly air and water, their volume will likely fall outside the measuring cup size. Also remember to limit salad dressings, which contain a lot of calories and fats.

How the LAP-BAND May Be Defeated:

- Drinking during meals
- Eating liquid or semisolid foods
- High calorie/fat snacks between meals (chips, sweets, and too many nuts or "junk" foods)
- Grazing
- Not exercising regularly
- Not maintaining follow-up with your bariatric center and having Band adjustments
- Taking 90 minutes to eat a large meal
- High calorie sauces

Complications

Sometimes the problems you are having are related to the Band. We refer to these problems as complications. Your surgeon will discuss these risks with you as part of informed consent. (See Chapter 11.)

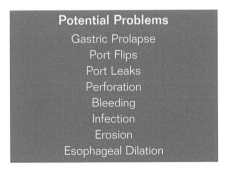

Potential Problems
Gastric Prolapse
Port Flips
Port Leaks
Perforation
Bleeding
Infection
Erosion
Esophageal Dilation

▼▼▼

Exercise and Physical Activity: The Keys to Burning Calories and Improving Your Health

Daniel Rooks, Ph.D.

You probably have heard many times that managing your weight is directly related to the number of calories you consume through eating and drinking and the number of those calories your body uses up during the day's activities. Unused calories are stored as body fat. A nice way of visualizing this concept of energy balance is to use a balance scale, with calories taken into the body on one side and calories burned by the body on the other.

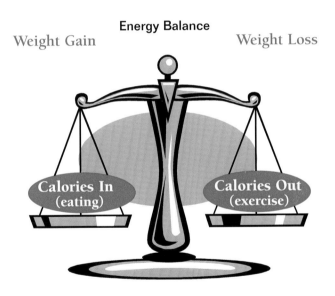

Energy Balance

Weight Gain   Weight Loss

Calories In (eating)   Calories Out (exercise)

While the LAP-BAND is an important tool to help limit the number of calories a person consumes, it affects only one side of the balance (calories in). Therefore, to lose weight faster, maintain the weight loss, improve your health, and enjoy more of life, you need to include ways to burn more calories each day (calories out). The good news here is that because you are in control of this aspect of managing your health, you have many options to choose from and can change your schedule anytime you wish. The key to successful weight management is to do something to burn extra calories every day. This chapter will describe the different ways you can do this and how to start and maintain a more active lifestyle, including an exercise program, to help you maximize your weight loss with the LAP-BAND and improve your health.

Burning Calories

There are three ways to burn calories and use up energy—metabolism, non-exercise body movement, and purposeful body movement. Often the largest amount of energy is used by the body to maintain its many functions. Thinking, the heart pumping blood throughout the body, digesting food, and other activities that go on in your body all require energy. This use of energy is referred to as your "metabolism." Muscle tissue is one of the biggest users of energy. The metabolism can be increased by the amount of muscle you have and how you use your muscles. The more you use them, the more physically fit you are, the more energy your metabolism uses up each day. In addition to metabolism is the energy your body uses during non-exercise movements. These movements can be conscious or unconscious and include fidgeting, repetitively moving your leg during sitting, tapping your foot, and other similar activities.

The most effective and most common way of burning calories is moving your body in daily activities. This body movement is referred to as physical activity. Physical activity can take many forms. Getting out of bed in the morning, showering, getting dressed, walking to your car and from the car to a store, doing yard work and house work, and lifting and carrying groceries all burn calories and all count as physical activity. The more effort an activity requires or the longer an activity lasts increases the number of calories burned during the activity. Remember, any body movement (physical activity) burns calories! Often used to mean the same thing, physical activity and exercise are different. While physical activity is any movement of the body, exercise is planned physical activity that improves your fitness—aerobic endurance, muscle strength, and flexibility—and your balance.

Benefits of Physical Activity and Exercise

There are many health-related benefits of adding physical activity to your daily routine and including several days of exercise each week. The most important benefits of these activities for the person having LAP-BAND surgery is increasing weight loss, maintaining muscle mass, and improving physical and emotional health. If you walk for 30 minutes and use another 150 calories each day from other activities, you will be burning about 300 calories daily from being physically active.

If you burn 300 calories more than you consume each day, you will lose 1 pound of body fat about every 12 days. Maintain this calorie balance for most of a year, and this translates to a loss of approximately 30 pounds. The physical activity, exercise, and the LAP-BAND can be a powerful combination to help a person lose weight.

The other major benefit from physical activity and exercise is the effect on muscle and other body systems. When you are more physically active, your muscles become better able to handle sugar in the blood (glucose tolerance). This is very important to the many individuals with diabetes or pre-diabetes. Also, when people are more physically active, they tend to be happier, feel better about themselves, are more optimistic, tend to eat better, not smoke, have more energy, and think more clearly. In addition to the immediate benefit of burning calories and helping with weight loss, research has shown that consistent physical activity and exercise are crucial for keeping weight off once it is lost. Long-term benefits of physical activity include better living with chronic conditions such as arthritis, asthma, and heart and lung disease and a reduced risk of diabetes, osteoporosis, physical disability, and dying from a heart attack or other cause.

How To Be More Physically Active

One of the most difficult challenges of becoming more physically active and starting an exercise program is knowing what to do and how often do it. The remaining sections will discuss these central issues.

It is recommended that people be more physically active 5 to 6 days a week. With a little creativity, you can figure out how to add physical activity into your personal life. When you go food shopping, use the cart for support and walk up and down every aisle, regardless of whether you need something from the aisle. When you get home, carry fewer bags of groceries at one time and make more trips from outside to your kitchen. You can park farther away from a store's entrance and walk the distance. If you use an elevator, walk up one flight of stairs then take the elevator the rest of the way. As you get fit, walk two flights then three or more. In time, you may be able to walk the entire way. Don't use the automatic door opener. Pushing or pulling a door open burns important calories. House and yard work are a good way to burn calories. Do you like to garden? Digging in the dirt, planting and tending flowers or vegetables, mowing the lawn, trimming bushes or trees are all good ways to burn calories and get the benefit of being outdoors and having an active hobby. You may want to join a local club or group where you can meet other people with similar interests. Stuck inside your home or apartment building? You can walk along hallways and climb stairs while listening to music. Set a goal of adding a new way of increasing physical activity to your schedule each week. When you run out of ideas, ask a friend or your family to help think of new ways to fit more physical activity into your day.

Starting and Maintaining an Exercise Program

Are you one of the many people who think exercise has to be done at a gym where everyone wears spandex, looks like a ballerina, and knows how to perform every exercise correctly on fancy-looking machines that make you sweat profusely? If you are, there is good news. A safe and effective exercise program for the person having LAP-BAND surgery or another weight loss surgery can be performed in the privacy of your own home or in a group at a community center with people of all levels of fitness, with similar health issues and exercise experience. Instructional videos, books, or group classes are available to help the person who is not familiar with exercise safely begin and maintain an exercise program.

An exercise program should be planned to meet each person's individual likes and dislikes, needs, and goals for maximum safety and effectiveness. When you develop your program, each exercise should follow the FITT-P guideline.

Frequency refers to how often the activity should be performed.

Intensity is the level of effort exerted to perform the exercise. Moderate intensity is sufficient to successfully manage weight, maintain muscle mass, and gain the many health benefits mentioned earlier.

Type of exercise refers to what exercise you perform, i.e., walking, cycling, swimming, hand weights, and machine-based exercises.

Time is how much time you perform aerobic exercises and how many repetitions you perform with strength training activities.

Progression refers to how to increase the amount of exercise performed to continue to improve fitness.

Before starting any exercise program, check with your primary care physician and weight loss surgeon as well as any other health care professional you see regularly, to make sure the program is appropriate for you. Remember, you don't have to wait until after surgery to begin exercising. In our program, we feel very strongly that exercise before and after surgery gives people the best chance for success. To demonstrate how an exercise program is developed, the following sections include a general program most people could follow.

The right amount of exercise will make you feel great and give you the best chance to succeed in your goals of losing body fat and maintaining a healthy weight. Too much exercise can make your muscles very sore and tired and increase the risk of injury. Too little exercise can lead to a loss of interest because you don't see the expected improvement in fitness.

Aerobic Exercise

Many people like walking because it is an important part of everyday life, and we will use walking in the example here. It is recommended that aerobic exercise be performed 3 to 5 times per week. Monitoring intensity can be done without high technology that measures your heart beat, although you can use this if you wish. A general rule is that you should walk (or perform any other aerobic activity) with a "purpose." If you cannot carry on a conversation while exercising, you are pushing too hard and should slow down a bit so you are able to finish your sentences. The intensity of exercise also can be monitored by measuring heart rate. The training heart rate—heart rate during exercise—is determined by your age and level of fitness.

Training heart rate for someone who has not exercised regularly **= (220 – Age) x .5 and .6**

Example of a 45-year-old person who is sedentary:

(220 – 45) x .5 = 175 x .5 = 88 beats per minute

(220 – 45) x .6 = 175 x .6 = 105 beats per minute

This 45-year-old person should have a heart rate between 88 and 105 beats per minute while exercising.

Choosing your exercise is a matter of personal preference; pick something you enjoy doing. The starting time is flexible, because many people having weight loss surgery can't walk for more than 10 minutes without stopping to rest. A person should begin walking for as long as he or she is comfortable. In our example, the person can start by walking for 10 minutes three times per day. The person can stop any time to rest. It is important to walk the full 10 minutes each time. In Week 2, the time can be increased by 1 minute (to 11 minutes) three times a day. Continue to add 1 to 2 minutes each week until walking for 30 minutes two to three times a day. Progression of 1 to 2 minutes ensures that the increase is not too large and that the person's body will be able to adapt to the increase in exercise.

Strength Training

Strength training exercise should be performed two to three times per week with at least 48 hour's rest between workouts. Strength training exercise can be done on the same day or different days of the week as aerobic exercise. Intensity for strength training exercise is determined by how much effort is given to performing the exercise movement. For the person preparing for or recovering from LAP-BAND surgery, a moderate intensity is sufficient to increase muscle tone and strength. A person should be able to complete the exercise without holding his or her breath. Strength training exercise is measured by the number of times an exercise is performed without resting. Performing an exercise a single time is referred to as a repetition and a series of repetitions performed one after the other is a set. Start with one set of 6 to 8 repetitions adding one or two repetitions each week. One or two sets of 8 to 12 repetitions of an exercise is sufficient. Exercises that involve the major muscles of the body should be included in an exercise program. Start with one or two exercises and add one exercise every 2 to 3 weeks as you feel comfortable. A program of six to eight exercises works well. In our example, we will include two basic exercises that are a good place to start. If you have soreness or pain with normal movements, check with your physician before trying the two movements.

Exercise Name and Technique

> **Chair squat** – sitting on the front half of a sturdy chair, stand up and sit down (one repetition). Repeat.

> **Side arm raises** – sitting in a chair or standing up behind a chair, start with arms resting at your sides. Smoothly move arms out to the side and toward over the head. Inhale as arms are raised and exhale as they are lowered. Stop when hands are at the highest point comfortably possible. Slowly lower to the starting position (one repetition). Repeat.

Flexibility

Flexibility exercises can be performed daily and should be done at least 4 to 5 days each week. The purpose of the exercises is to increase the comfort range of movement in major joints—neck, shoulders, back, arms, hips, knees and ankles. Flexibility exercises, also called stretching, should be done in a relaxed and gentle manner. Exercise selection and instruction can be found with a group class, video or book. A choice of exercises can be made with the assistance of a physical therapist or qualified fitness professional. Movements should be held for 15 to 30 seconds and repeated twice.

Resources

Examples of appropriate exercises can be found in materials offered by the Arthritis Foundation, the American Heart Association, American Diabetes Association, and other similar organizations. A book that describes basic exercises with pictures and words is *The Everyday Arthritis Solution* published by Reader's Digest. Ask your doctor, nurse, and physical therapist about good exercises to add to your program. Also, many group exercise classes offer instruction on basic and advanced exercise movements.

Summary

When you decide to have LAP-BAND surgery, you make a major life decision to lose weight and improve your health. However, surgery is only one part of that decision. How you care for yourself before and after surgery will ultimately determine how successful you are at losing weight, keeping the weight off, and improving your health and your life. We believe that being more physically active before and after surgery is very important to the success of the weight loss surgery patient. This chapter described the benefits of physical activity and exercise and how to include the needed amounts into your busy week. It is not easy, but with some creative thinking on your part, it is possible to be more physically active each day and consistently include enjoyable exercise activities that improve your physical and emotional health and well-being. The key to successful weight management is to do something to burn extra calories every day. Every minute of physical activity counts!

▼▼▼
Troubleshooting the BAND

Occasionally, Band patients think, "What is wrong? Why is this thing not working?" If this occurs to you or someone close to you, first make sure that nothing *is* wrong with the Band or its placement. Your surgeon can probably confirm or easily make sure that everything is okay. This is one reason why a regular visit with your bariatric center is important. Patients who fail to follow-up with the center will commonly not lose, or will even gain, weight.

The BAND is Not Working?

Many times, when a person thinks, "The BAND is not working," it actually is working. For most people on course with the program, the target weight loss is one to two pounds a week. That means that 4 to 5 pounds a month is right on target. You need to remember that you are in this for the long run. If you had your Band placed around the same time as a friend who had a gastric bypass, it can be frustrating. The bypass patient can lose 100 pounds in the first several months. You just need to keep in mind that you are losing weight in a healthy and potentially durable fashion. Just stay the course. *Remember the story of the tortoise and the hare?* In published studies at 3 to 5 years, the weight loss with a Band or bypass can be comparable.

If a patient is truly not losing weight when the Band is placed and adjusted well, there are several factors that must be examined. The most frequent reason the Band is not working has to do with the person who is using this tool, the patient. They may have received inadequate training or counseling in its use or forgotten lessons learned. The program can be defeated. Your bariatric center is there with you to make sure that it does work. Ask them.

When Eating Is Painful.

If you dread sitting down to the table to eat because it is painful, something is probably wrong. Maybe the *adjustment is too tight*. Ironically, patients with too tight an adjustment can actually gain weight. This is because eating solid food is how the Band functions best. If the Band is too tight, solid food may not be able to pass at all. If you are spitting back up all solid food all the time, your body will naturally gravitate toward eating high-calorie, high-fat foods, such as milk shakes, cakes, pies and creams. Such foods, which pass more easily through the Band, will be absorbed normally, and you can actually gain weight. This can be hard to grasp when you are spitting up anything solid, but it is the case.

If your Band adjustment is such that you can usually keep down solid food, then the answer is more likely the *quantity of food* you are eating. This is actually the most frequent cause of Band failure and pain. The Band creates a constriction around the top part of the stomach, which produces a pouch of stomach above the Band. When this pouch is filled with a small amount of solid food that is delayed from passing through by the constriction of the Band, the stomach is full, and you feel comfortably restricted. If, however, you take another bite of food after the stomach pouch is full, or take a drink, that next swallow will have to stay in the esophagus (food pipe). The esophagus does not like food to stay there. The esophagus will start to contract and spasm to move the food out. This can be very uncomfortable. Each person experiences different sensations. It may feel as if something is stuck in your throat. It can feel like chest or back pain. It may make you spit the food back up or just sit there and make you feel uncomfortable.

Food in stomach pouch = satisfied

Once this "bite too much," or let's call it "bite *X*," is taken, the options are few and are all a compromise. Drinking a liquid at this point might help the food pass, or it might not. If the liquid does move the food through, you will not only absorb all the food you have pushed through, but now your pouch will be empty and you will need to eat more. Alternatively, the additional liquid may make you spit everything up. If you do spit it up, you will keep approximately a third of the calories you ate and, again, your pouch will be empty, and you will need to eat more. This pattern of overeating and spitting up can be very ineffective and also may be associated with chronic dilation of your stomach pouch and/or herniation or movement of the Band.

Food in esophagus = discomfort

Some patients just leave it there and may feel uncomfortable for a long time. The idea of having the Band is to make you feel comfortable, not uncomfortable. In these cases, this tool is simply not being used properly. This is like using the wrong end of a hammer or using a drill spinning in the wrong direction.

The way to correct this is by **not** taking *bite X* that gets stuck in your esophagus. This may sound simple, but sometimes it is not. You see, when you decide to take that one "bite too much," *bite X*, the previous bite may not have made it to your stomach yet. Even if the previous bite had made it, it may not have signaled to your brain that you are full. The best way is for you to remember how many bites you can take of this food at this time of day. The nice thing is that you don't have to figure it out by tomorrow, next week, or even by next month. You are going to have the Band for years. You have time to do little experiments along the way to find out what is most comfortable. Comfort is the key. If it is not comfortable, you won't be able to make it work for years.

The Criminal Foods

A different group of foods, unlike the ones we just spoke about, are foods that are not held up by the Band, but pass right through instead. Some of these can be high in calories and fat such as sweets, chips, nuts, and alcohol. These foods are *the common criminals.* Some of them can single-handedly defeat our program. A partial list of these *criminals* is shown in below. There are many more foods that are not included.

Foods That Pass Through the Band	
Cheese puffs	Ice cream
Chocolate	Pasta alfredo
Milk shakes	Instant breakfast drinks
Cheese and cheese dips	Smoothies

Removing these culprits from your diet, your kitchen, your house, and your work could quickly troubleshoot problems you're having with the Band. The dietitian can work with you by creating a food log like the one included at the end of the book.

▼▼▼ Frequently Asked Questions

Weight loss with a LAP-BAND brings new experiences to eating and living. These experiences will be unique to each person going through this new adventure. Certain questions are common and frequent. Having these questions answered is important and is one of the important reasons to follow-up with your bariatric center on a regular basis after your Band is placed. Here are some of the most frequent questions we encounter.

"Why is it more difficult to swallow in the morning than in the evening? I can barely get water down in the morning, and I can eat anything I want at night."

This is a very common finding in Band patients. The exact reason for this is not currently known. It could be as simple as some swelling in the stomach wall, like puffy eyes. Maybe it is the result of saliva or stomach secretions overnight. It could be a result of the condition of your stomach in the morning. Your stomach is a big muscle used to grind up food. The Band places a rigid plastic ring around the top of the stomach. If you can imagine placing a rigid ring around your upper arm, the ring would be loose if your arm is straight and very tight if you bent your arm to make a muscle. The size of the stomach opening through the Band is going to completely depend on your stomach's current state of contraction. If the stomach is relaxed, the opening is large, and food travels easily through the Band. If the stomach is forcefully contracting, the opening through the Band will be small, and food or liquid will have a more difficult time getting through the stomach.

Many patients will find that they get some relief in the morning by taking some warm liquid like tea or coffee. This warm temperature can help relax the stomach and allow things to slide through better. Likewise, you may find that cold water or juice will make it worse. Each patient must find what works best for him or her, since no two people are the same. But don't be alarmed if sometimes you can eat a whole plate of food and other times you can barely get down water. Nothing is wrong or broken.

"Sometimes if I eat something like chicken or bread, I cannot swallow even water afterwards and spit up everything. What is going on?"

Some foods may consistently be so delayed passing through the Band opening that food will temporarily be blocked off. The exact foods that cause this will vary from person to person. It is an important process for you to discover which foods work and which do not. The foods that go through the slowest can be your best friend, because you need the least amount of them to feel full. The size of the stomach opening through a well-adjusted Band is approximately the size of a ballpoint pen. Hard objects that are larger than this can potentially block the opening. Large pills, for example, need to be broken in half or quarters to prevent them from blocking the stomach. Be sure to read the labels on your medications. Some extended-release tablets must not be broken up. These may have to be changed to regular-duration tablets and taken more frequently during the day.

Always try to chew your food so that all the pieces you swallow are smaller than a pencil eraser. You may want to count the number of chews (25) or use a rubber-tip baby spoon to teach yourself to take small bites. An egg timer or hour glass can help you slow the speed of eating. Waiting 1 to 2 minutes between bites is a good start. You will need to find out what food, bite size, and interval works best for you. If you get the sensation that you are blocked, give the food or medicine time to pass. If you are uncomfortable, try sipping some warm liquids. This may relax your stomach and allow the food to pass. If you begin to forcefully vomit, rather than just spitting up, you may need to call your physician. Forceful vomiting can cause your stomach to herniate up through your Band. This could cause the stomach to completely block off and the stomach wall to be injured as well. If this is persistent for several hours, you may need to have fluid removed from the Band to relieve the obstruction. Call your surgeon.

It is an important process to discover which solid foods work for you. We want you to tolerate solid foods so that the pouch remains full following meals. If you can take only liquids and cannot take any solid food, then your Band may be too tight. This will ironically cause you to fail to lose, or even to gain, weight. Remember, if you are taking only liquids, the pouch will not fill, and then you will be hungry. As a result, you will eat (or drink) more than if your adjustment was correct.

"Will I be able to feel the Band in there?"

You will not be able to feel the plastic ring around your stomach. The outside surface of your stomach does not have the specific nerves that would allow you to sense its location on your stomach. You will be able to feel the effects of the Band by the way it controls the food passing through your stomach. This sensation varies from person to person. The "restriction," as many people call it, can be sensed anywhere from your throat to your upper abdomen. Sometimes patients describe a pressure while swallowing or fullness in the upper abdomen while the food passes into the stomach. You will have to learn how the restriction feels in your case. Prior to the first several Band adjustments, many patients have no sensation at all. Because everyone's stomach is a different size, and the Band comes in only a couple of sizes, it could require several fills before you can sense that the Band is there. Do not be worried if you have no sensation of the Band at all after it is initially placed; it's there. The primary feeling you will have is a decrease in hunger.

Many, but not all, people can feel the adjustment port, which lies underneath the skin of your upper abdomen. Sometimes people think what they feel under the skin is the Band. The port, which lies on top of your belly wall muscle, under the skin, is separate from the Band around the stomach. A long, thin, flexible tube that is more than a foot long connects the two parts. If something bumps or irritates the port under the skin, it is a long way from the Band.

In some people, the subcutaneous port can be uncomfortable following surgery. This is the largest incision, which will result in the most swelling and will require the most healing after your operation. In patients who lose a great deal of weight, the subcutaneous port could start to be noticeable as a bump under the skin. Occasionally, this port will need to be repositioned. This is usually a short, same-day outpatient procedure.

"When does the Band need to be removed?"

There is no date when the Band must be removed, and we expect that most patients will keep it for a lifetime. The groups in Australia have patients who have had the Band in place for more than 10 years. The materials that make up the Band will last for a long time. The stomach and other parts of your body that come in contact with the Band will form what we call a capsule around the plastic. This capsule is made up of scar tissue, which your body uses to separate itself from any foreign material inside it. The materials used in the Band are the same materials that have been used in many other implantable medical devices for decades and have been proven to be safe long-term.

Think about the Band like an artificial knee joint. That type of implant typically lasts 10 to 15 years. Bands, which need to be repositioned, can often be replaced with new Bands in a slightly different position. Another nice feature is that if a Band system doesn't work for a patient for any particular reason, the patient can be converted to a different weight-loss procedure, such as a gastric bypass. You don't really burn any bridges with Band placement compared to other weight-loss procedures that re-route the gastrointestinal tract.

"What happens to the Band after I have lost my weight?"

The Band is a great maintenance tool. There are no data for which the Band must be removed. Patients are able to maintain or continue to lose weight safely if they remain on the program. The common reasons for removing the Band are typically for care of complications, which are fortunately becoming much less frequent. Potential complications include Band erosions, slippage, pouch dilation, and port problems.

It is likely that sometime, in the not too distant future, there will be a medication that can relieve hunger and make the Band unnecessary. Unfortunately, this type of medication will not be available very soon, at least to our knowledge. Fortunately, having the Band in place leaves your body in its normal anatomic configuration. Even if a medical cure for hunger came out the week after your Band was placed, you could be returned to your near-normal state relatively quickly and easily. This is not the case if you have had other weight-loss operations. Reversibility is one of the attributes of Band surgery.

"I don't seem to be losing very much weight right now, less than a pound a week. My clothes size seems to be shrinking though."

It is common for Band patients to reach a plateau where they are replacing excess body weight with lean body mass or muscle. This process of replacing fat with muscle will result in a visual change in your appearance that exceeds your observed weight loss on the scale. Muscle is a heavier tissue than fat so more muscle can be carried in a given space than fat. Having more muscle will accelerate your weight loss since every ounce of muscle requires energy to work. As you will recall, your loss is a combination of both decreased calories taken in and the increased calories used up. Having more muscle will always be a good thing. So keep with it.

"Why can't I drink sodas?"

The carbonation in soda does not work well with the Band. If you drink a soda, the fluid can pass quickly through the upper stomach pouch and Band into the lower part of your stomach. If you have difficulty belching due to the Band constriction, the expanding gas from the carbonation will be trapped between the Band and the outlet valve of your stomach, so the bubbles have no place to go. This causes what is called gastric distension, which can be very uncomfortable. In addition, this could change the position of the Band on the stomach. The position of the band is critical to its function. Other patients report the feeling of the carbonated soda staying above the band in the pouch and expanding. The bottom line is that many sodas tend to be very high in calories, and diet soda is a slippery slope to regular soda.

If you are a person who is addicted to diet soda, here is a trick: just take a two-liter bottle and partially open the top. Place it in the refrigerator and allow the carbonation to escape. Then you could safely have your diet soda, or wean yourself, since it rarely tastes as good without bubbles.

"What about alcohol?"

Beer has carbonation, so that makes it a bad choice. Although Paul O'Brien has published one study showing that a glass of red wine enhances weight loss, alcohol is discouraged because it tends to be high in calories. Everything that passes your lips needs to be considered in the balance. Our goal is to choose liquids that are low in calories. And always stay away from liquids during meals. This will wash the food right out of the pouch, and it will get absorbed right away, and you will still be hungry because the pouch will be empty!

"Will I have lots of floppy skin after I lose the weight?"

It is hard to know who will have a problem with excess skin after weight loss. Just like predicting which women will have stretch marks after childbirth, all people respond a little differently to the same weight loss. Obviously, patients who start from very high weights, say greater than 400 pounds, and lose a large portion of their excess body weight will have the greatest potential for excess skin.

It is important to be patient after you start to lose weight when considering removing excess skin. We strongly discourage any procedure on your skin during the first 2 years after Band placement or when you are getting close to an ideal body weight. If you have a procedure to tighten the skin under your arms or abdomen after losing 50 pounds and then you lose 50 more, you may still have the original problem. Plastic surgery can be very helpful, but it also can be very expensive. Cosmetic surgery will generally not be covered by your health insurance.

Some patients have asked if they might donate their excess skin to a burn center and perhaps offset the cost of surgery. Unfortunately, burn centers do not accept skin from such a source.

After you have reached a stable weight that you are comfortable with, your surgeon or primary care physician can recommend a plastic surgeon to speak with you. He or she will best be able to tell you what procedures are available and what to expect. It is not a problem to have your abdominal skin worked on by the plastic surgeon. The port under your skin can be left in place or moved by the bariatric surgeon at the time of plastic surgery. There is also a low-profile port available if your port sticks out too much. Make sure that your Band surgeon knows what is going on with your port. Access and adjustment of the Band via your subcutaneous port is always important.

▼▼▼
A Little Pep Talk and Testimonials

Frequently, after someone has had a Band for a while, he or she could use a little pep talk. One of the fundamental principles of the Band is that weight loss is slow and natural. This is a great feature because it is healthy and sustainable, but it is possible to get a little anxious. Even if you are on course with the program, your adjustment is good, and you are losing weight, the progress can seem slow. But remember that the target rate of loss is 1 to 2 pounds a week. This translates to maybe only 4 pounds a month. This amount may not seem very glamorous or impressive but it can result in more than 100 pounds lost over 2 years and more than 150 pounds lost over 3 years.

This loss of extra fat will be sustainable and easy to maintain. There will not be a need to measure your vitamin and other blood levels all the time, because you are hooked up as you always were and will not be malabsorbing what you do eat. Unless there is a problem, it will not even be necessary to check your Band. You just need to stay the course and enjoy not being an obese person. You should enjoy walking, running, or doing the other things you couldn't do the year before.

Many people with a Band in place lose much of the desire to eat at all and have to constantly remind themselves to eat. Others can get tired of not being able to eat certain foods that they always loved.

Many Band patients will say that there will always be some food that you will have to "give up" following each adjustment or tightening of your Band. This may not necessarily be true. Try a little experiment. Although the size of the stomach pouch above the Band is small, there is stomach there. The opening between that pouch and the rest of the stomach should be about the size of a pencil eraser when the Band is at a good adjustment. For meats, you may have to cut the pieces that small prior to chewing. If you chew your food up to a size smaller than a pencil eraser, you should be able to eat it. It will be the *amount* that you will need to change. Certain meats and breads tend to be difficult for many Band patients. Very frequently it will seem that right after you start eating one of these foods, it will get stuck, cause pressure, and want to come back up. Don't give up on these foods; these foods could be your best friends. These foods, which are held up longer by the constriction in the Band, will keep the pouch of stomach above the Band filled the longest. You will therefore require less food to stay satisfied for the day.

Testimonials

We believe that it is very important to speak with past patients about the LAP-BAND. Why did they decide to have the weight-loss surgery? Why did they choose the Band rather than gastric bypass? What were their major concerns? What was the process like? Did they have complications or problems adjusting? And the major question—would they do it again?

To help our readers, we asked our patients at support groups to write one page each about their experiences. We accepted all testimonials without being selective. Again, we don't want to sugarcoat the process. Although rare, patients can die from an operation. More commonly, patients may need an operation to repair or revise the Band afterwards. But for most patients in our practice, patients can lose weight and improve quality of life. These are the personal comments they wanted shared with you.

▼▼▼

Week One:

I had my surgery on a Monday. Everything went great and I came out without a problem. But I was in a lot of pain. It didn't hurt so much where they had made the incisions for the surgical instruments, but I was very sore where they had inserted the port (the access tube that allows doctors to tighten the band by injecting saline, further promoting a full feeling). It is on my left side just above my belly button. The incision was a couple of inches long, and the port is stitched into the muscle. They gave me some pain medication, and that helped some. The next morning I went down for a test called a barium swallow. They gave me a really disgusting clear drink first. I somehow got that down. Then I had the barium swallow to make sure everything inside was working properly. Then they started me on some water, which you must drink from a medicine cup, and they started me on Carnation Instant Breakfast drink.

I expected to get out of the hospital that day, but I was getting queasy going from x-ray back to my room. The hospital staff didn't want to take any chances in case I was coming down with a virus or something. I was better by Wednesday and left the hospital.

Over the next few days, I continued with the water, Carnation Instant Breakfast drink and added some other protein drinks, some flavored, some not. I was amazed that I would drink just a little and would feel very full. I just didn't want anything more!!

I did feel somewhat depressed in that first week. It was hard to get around. I'm used to being busy, working and running after my kids. And I was very sore. I remember thinking, is this ever going to go away? Will I ever sleep on my side, my stomach or be able to pick up my baby again? You know in your brain that it will get better, but it was hard to think that way at first. I needed to use a cough pillow to get comfortable enough to sleep. But each day I felt 100% better than the day before.

Weeks Two & Three:

Exactly 1 week after having the surgery, I went back to work. I had tried driving the day before and it felt okay. I don't have a lot of heavy lifting in my job (I run a small law office) and I had been really bored. After I got to the office, I was uncomfortable (still very sore) and washed out. It was the most I had done in a week, and this was major surgery! My body was still getting rid of toxins and I hadn't had solid food in a week. You're depending upon your vitamins and protein drinks for strength. I did make it through that day, and picked up my daughter from dance.

I was able to drink other liquids—soup broths, milk. But quite honestly, after 2 weeks I had had enough of that. You're supposed to stay on liquids only for 4 weeks but I cheated, and anyone who tells you they don't cheat is lying! I needed texture. So I started testing it. I threw some canned chicken into the food processor, and I ate about one tablespoon with no problems. I still stuck to soups and cottage cheese, but everything else went into the food processor!

Week Four:

I got the green light to start on Stage 4 of my recovery. That means I could eat scrambled hamburger, eggs—moist things. I made Shake and Bake Pork Chops for the family and cut it up like I was a toddler learning how to eat. Just a few bites and I felt like I had eaten two entire chops, with stuffing and corn! Your stomach does growl and you do get hungry during the day, but just a little bit of anything fills you right up. I would eat one meatball for lunch and I was really full.

I was still a bit sore, but could sleep on my side and stomach! All my wounds had healed and I could finally pick up my baby!

Week Five:

Since my surgery, I have lost 21 pounds. I've started exercising—1/2 mile each day on my treadmill and about 5 to 10 minutes of stretching and weight training. I am completely pain free and feel great!!!

Would I do it again? Yup. I would. If it's 2 weeks of discomfort for a lifetime of health, I would take it any day.

PS: The pants I wore before surgery are now way too big for me. I tried to wear them the other day, and they kept sliding down!

▼▼▼

I would like to thank two very important people in my life without whom I could not have done this; first my wonderful wife, who supported me and stood by me from the beginning, and Dr. Daniel Jones, who saved and changed my life. Without them I don't think I would be alive today.

My name is Joel and I am 59 years old. I've been a master chef for approximately 30 years. I have been overweight most of my adult life and have had a lot of different medical problems, such as being diabetic—taking insulin three times per day and severe pain in both legs from carrying around all the extra weight. Some days the pain was so bad I could not even walk. I also suffered from sleep apnea requiring a special machine with a mask to assist my breathing so I could sleep. As the years went by, my problems just got worse. Being a chef and around food 12 hours a day made it very difficult for me to diet. I tried many different diets, lost weight and gained it back numerous times. I was at the end of my rope. If I didn't do something very quickly I would probably die.

I had heard about gastric bypass and called Beth Israel Deaconess Medical Center. They sent me information to review, and after I did, I made the call to set up an appointment to see if I could have the surgery. I didn't even tell my wife at this time. I would say, "I have a doctor's appointment at such and such a time" and she would say, "no," because, you see, she always made all my doctor appointments. But this I did myself. I wanted to see if this procedure was right for me. I went to the hospital, completed the forms, and had a lot of questions. I had a physical, saw a nurse, a psychiatrist, and a doctor to see if the bypass was for me. The psychiatrist asked me why I wanted this done. I told her I had a weight problem and other medical issues and I just wanted to bring my food intake down to lose weight. She then told me about a new kind of stomach procedure that would make me eat less and told me that I was an excellent candidate for this new procedure called a gastric LAP-BAND. She told me more about it, and I told her this was just for me, and God was watching over me. I agreed to do it.

It took a few months of paperwork and doctor visits before the surgery. Then I told my wife what I had planned to do. She thought I was crazy, but I told her this was my last resort. I took her to orientation where a group of people like me shared their stories. We met one of the other surgeons. It was supposed to be Dr. Jones, but he was called away that night. My wife told me after the meeting "I'm with you all the way, honey". A couple of days later I had my date for surgery, August 21, 2003—the day Dr. Jones changed my life. Up to that point I had never met Dr. Jones. The morning of my surgery I was waiting in my room, people coming in and getting me ready—anesthesiologists, nurses, etc., checking me over and asking me different questions. Then all of a sudden someone came in my room and said "Hello, Mr. Sisel." I said, "Who the heck are you?" He said, "I'm Dr. Jones" and I said, "No, you're not—You are the elusive Dr. Jones."

I felt very comfortable with Dr. Jones doing my surgery. The surgery went perfectly. I have five small incisions in my abdomen and a portal under my skin in the abdomen so Dr. Jones can adjust the size of the Band by injecting saline to make it larger or smaller. I was up and walking 2 hours after the surgery and went home the next day. The next few weeks after the surgery were the hardest for me. The liquid protein diet did not agree with me, so, being a chef, I changed my diet a little to better agree with me. I changed it to a light chicken broth with a little rice, and I was okay. Then things started to change. I started losing weight, feeling better, and adjusted to eating differently, and the weight started coming off. I started to change. It's been over 3 years since my surgery. I feel good and I look great. I lost 14 inches on my waist and over 100 pounds at my greatest loss. I take pride in my appearance; I have self esteem again. I am different inside and out since I lost my weight. Heavy people are treated differently than others and are looked down upon. I recommend this procedure with all my heart and soul, but remember that it's not a magic pill. You need to work at it every single day. When I had my surgery, the only person I told was my wife. I did not tell my friends, people at work, or family. I had my surgery during my 2-week vacation. After the surgery I told my son and my daughter what I had done. I just can't say enough about this procedure. I've been on the radio, the Internet, and was included in a DVD about this procedure. I highly recommend it to everyone; it's a lifesaver.

My wife and I were all dressed up at a formal event. The hostess came over and said to my wife, Cheryl, "It is so great to see you, but where is Joel?" I was standing right next to her, but the hostess didn't even recognize me. It is such a great feeling. People who have known me for years don't even recognize me. Starting from day one with the receptionists to the nurses, to the doctors and everyone affiliated with the LAP-BAND I was treated with utmost dignity and respect, and that is a great feeling.

I love Dr. Jones for saving my life and saving my wife's life, which is a whole other story. I used to eat a four-pound chicken in 10 minutes. I ate not because I was hungry, but just to eat. Now if I eat a chicken thigh I am full, which tells you how much things have changed. Before the operation I was obsessed with food—eat, eat, eat—now, food is no longer important to me. I eat only if I'm hungry—three small meals a day and I enjoy them greatly. If I'm not hungry I just don't eat. I no longer eat just to eat. The small space in my stomach is too important to me. Another reason I decided to have the surgery is to see my daughter get married and dance at her wedding.

My wife, Cheryl, also has a very special bond with Dr. Jones. Approximately 2 1/2 years ago she was diagnosed with a rare form of stomach cancer and needed surgery. She was very scared until she found out that Dr. Jones would be doing her surgery. She had the utmost confidence in him as a surgeon, and this is why we have the relationship that we do with Dr. Jones—a two-for-one special. When my wife found out she needed stomach surgery as soon as possible, Dr. Jones' schedule was full, but he said he would fit her in right away even if he had to sleep over in the hospital in his pajamas.

When I used to go in for my check-ups, I would bake and bring desserts for all the staff—homemade fudge, pies and cheesecakes, etc. to show my thanks. Dr. Jones said to me, "I have to stop this because if I keep it up, I would have to do the LAP-BAND on myself!"

One day I made lunch for the staff—assorted sandwiches and cakes. I found out Dr. Jones liked roast beef with mayonnaise. He told me that every time he ordered it he received funny looks because most people have it with mustard. So, I made him a two foot, cooked to perfection roast beef sandwich, three inches thick with lettuce and tomato, with many packages of mayonnaise around the sandwich. You should have seen his face. That night I got a call from his wife on my answering machine thanking me for supper that night.

A few weeks after my wife's surgery I had an appointment with Dr. Jones. He asked me how my wife was doing, and I replied, "Emotionally not so good." At that point, he stopped my appointment, asked me to wait outside the exam room, called my wife on the phone, and talked to her for about 20 minutes. Then he asked me to come back in and finish my appointment.

I had decided that when I finally reached my goal weight I wanted one thing, so I bought it. What was it? A complete leather outfit, including leather bike pants, vest, boots, jacket, gloves, and a special hat called a dew rag. My wife thought I was nuts. I also bought leather shorts for the summer, and a leather belt with a big silver buckle. I looked so good I scared myself. This is the kind of self-confidence I now have since I lost the weight.

After 11 years I lost my job due to budget cuts, but don't despair, because I found a new job even before I left the last one. I was a chef for a senior adult lunch program, which was in the same building as an assisted living program. When word reached the employees at the assisted living program, they came to me and asked me to run their two kitchens and manage the kitchen staff. Every day my wife would set out my clothes for me because I had to "dress the part." I was a food service director and had a staff of about 20 people plus 100 residents to feed. Every day I would wear a different outfit and go around to visit the residents to see how dinner went the night before. They would remark how good I looked because many of these people knew me before the Band. I had one staff person, a registered care nurse who would give me two thumbs up every day and say I looked great. That made me feel so great, words cannot describe.

As an orthodox Jew, every Saturday I go to temple to pray. I've been going to the same temple for about 20 years, so the other congregants saw the change in my weight. Typically I wore a shirt and tie to the synagogue, but on Purim, a holiday on which costumes may be worn, I told my wife that I was going to wear my biker outfit. When I walked into temple wearing my leather outfit, everyone was in shock, even the Rabbi. He came to me and said, "Which is the real Joel, the one who comes to temple in a suit and tie, or the one in the leather pants?" I leaned over to the Rabbi and whispered into his ear and said, "Rabbi, this is the real Joel."

I take great pride in the way I look now and how I feel about myself inside and out. My wife says, "Dr. Jones created a monster!"

▼▼▼

I was 66 years of age when I decided to have the surgery. I was relatively active, played golf, went to the gym. I am a retired physical education professor. I had lost over 100 pounds. Three times in my life. I was desperate. I was slowing down, not being able to function. I weighed 260 pounds.

My initial counseling meeting with "Ronna" (psychologist) was the most influential meeting of my entire life. She said, "You won't be better next year; it will be worse." I had to really pursue getting the LAP-BAND because of my age. I went to an orientation meeting, met Dr. Jones and convinced him I was a young 66-year-old woman. Three years prior, I had had bilateral knee replacements. If I could handle that, I could handle anything.

My LAP-BAND is my best friend. It tells me when it is enough. It is the built-in supreme diet pill. The Band around the stomach is not the only answer. The major work is done from the neck up. I have had no complications. I have lost 70 pounds. I had my surgery Dec. 5, 2005.

The decision to have the LAP-BAND was the best decision I have made in the last 30 years of my life. I feel reborn. I now walk on the golf course, no riding in a cart, and I work out three times a week in a gym. Thirty minutes cardio, 30 minutes weight resistance exercises, and once a week, I do core ball work with my trainer. I have met my physical goals of walking on the golf course, walking up the dune to my favorite beach, and wearing a size 16 pants. My diabetes medications are two-thirds gone. My hemoglobin A^{1c} is 5.6.

The most important lesson of all for me is to listen to the LAP-BAND. The Band constantly fights the beast in me. So far, the Band is winning. I can only do what I can this minute. I go to a support group out of the hospital once a week.

The only recommendation is to have more contact with the patients after surgery. Once every 2 months is not enough. Counseling weekly is needed. And not just for the first year, but forever.

Dr. Jones, his hands, and my Band are my savior. "Ronna" must play a more active role in the follow-up care. Her knowledge of the psychology of obesity must be better utilized for the patients to have long-term success.

▼▼▼

I have struggled with my weight since the birth of my children 12 years ago. My weight ballooned to 260 pounds. I knew I had to take action in order to have "quality of life" as I got older. I was tired, depressed, had high blood pressure—the list goes on and on... As most overweight individuals, I tried every diet known... from fen/fen to Jenny Craig®, Weight Watchers, etc. I would be successful in the short term and then gain the weight back with an additional 10 to 20 pounds. I began investigating weight loss surgery as my last resort. My cousin, who also had LAP-BAND surgery, and I began the weight loss seminar circuit. We first attended a seminar on gastric bypass. I was very interested in gastric bypass because it seemed like a guaranteed weight-loss surgery. I was, however, concerned about any surgery with a mortality rate. We then began to research LAP-BAND. We went to several seminars and researched the surgery rigorously via the Internet. When I made the decision to take control of my health, LAP-BAND was the solution that was right for me. It was less invasive, reversible, a short recovery period compared to gastric bypass, and historically patients were more successful in the long-term than gastric bypass.

I am a sales support manager for a major telecommunications company. I had my surgery in April, 2005, and within 17 months have lost 102 pounds. The secret to my success is the knowledge that the Band is only a tool and not a magic solution. The Band allows me to control my portion size, and it is punitive if I overeat (throwing up). My motto is "just because I can eat it, doesn't mean I should." I did not discover until 12 months into the "Band" that I could eat crunchy, junk type items (i.e., chips, crunchy chocolate). If I had known this immediately after surgery, I don't know if I would have been successful, because the tendency to continue to eat junk would have still been there immediately following surgery.

I did struggle the first 6 months with feeling deprived. My motto at that point, was "Just because I don't eat it, doesn't mean I don't WANT to." I was not one of the patients who never felt hunger. I was very hungry until my first fill 8 weeks after my surgery. I did still crave fast food, etc. Like I mentioned previously, the first 6 months for me were not fun, but more mentally than physically. Most overweight people don't eat because they are hungry, they eat out of emotion... it took me a while to come to grips with that knowledge and learn to manage it. I was probably a year post-op before I could honestly say I was glad that I had the surgery and would do it again. I know that several people are able to say that well before a year, but again, mine was a somewhat emotional journey.

I did not go to group support, but I did have my cousin who was 6 weeks ahead of me! The emotional support we have given to each other has played a HUGE part in my weight loss. She has been extremely successful with a 139 pound weight loss in 18 months!

All of that said, I am now successful because I feel very empowered about my food choices etc. Keep in mind, I've only had one fill and then had part of it removed. I do still have restriction but would certainly be able to eat more than a cup of food if I chose to. Most of the time, I choose not to! I manage to eat about 1,000 calories a day currently.

The obvious benefits, of feeling better, looking better, having more confidence, a longer life expectancy because of the weight loss. I am no longer treated for high blood pressure and high cholesterol, and of course, I am now much more physically and socially active due to the weight loss. This stems from feeling better and, of course, having greater self-esteem.

The only complication I had was that I had too much restriction after my first fill. That was easily fixed with an 'unfill.' Other than that, I have had no problems. Yes, I would have LAP-BAND again. I haven't really "enjoyed" the weight loss journey, but I have "enjoyed" the end-result.

I think the best candidates for LAP-BAND surgery are those who have had a long struggle with obesity but are not looking for a quick fix. Good candidates understand that the Band is a tool, not a miracle. They are willing to follow the rules and are scared to death about health issues. Ideally, they have a partner/friend who has also had surgery for support.

Poor candidates for LAP-BAND surgery are individuals who have only been obese for a short period of time. They think there is no effort expended on the part of the patient and don't understand that the lifestyle change is forever, not temporary. Individuals who are doing it only to "look" better, i.e., please a spouse, get a spouse and are not willing to commit emotionally as well as physically will not succeed. The surgery is the EASY part.

▼▼▼

My weight had been an issue for over 17 years. I knew I was not getting any younger. I have seen my parents and all the medicine they are on, I am sure, due to them being overweight. My weight had gotten so out of hand. I had to start on high blood pressure medicine. I had tried every diet, every diet pill and so-called plan. Enough was enough.

I am sitting all day and working on a computer. I had my surgery June 13, 2005, and in a little over a year I have lost 91 pounds.

Well, one thing that helps me is the fact I don't eat fast food. I can't eat fries, hamburgers, hot dogs, and I stay away from a lot of bread. I eat a lot of fish, chicken, veggies. Don't get me wrong, I have my moments and I do the chocolate thing, but overall I eat baked food. The one thing that also helps me is the chicken noodle soup and crackers I eat.

The benefits for me have been my health. I feel so much younger. I look younger and have more energy. The LAP-BAND has helped me control my hunger. I am not constantly hungry, and when I do eat, it is light food. I have had great success with the LAP-BAND surgery, and I have had no complications since my surgery. I was able to get off my blood pressure medicine, and the dosage on my thyroid medicine has been lowered twice now since my surgery.

I can take walks with my dogs and not get tired; I exercise more, walk up and down the stairs and not feel like I am going to pass out. I just have more strength and energy now with my weight loss.

Anyone who is around 100 pounds overweight and has health issues related to weight would be a good candidate for this surgery.

▼▼▼

I have had a weight problem all my adult life. And, yes, in those years I have tried just about every diet. Yes, they all worked and I lost weight, but those pounds always seemed to just keep coming back with added pounds usually. What I never realized is that I had an eating disorder that I would have to deal with for my entire life. As the years went by and I kept losing and regaining weight I just felt like I would have to get used to being "fat." (I hate that word)

When I lost my husband of 32 years to cancer in 1992, I really just seemed to give up. Now my life was going to work, eating at a buffet every lunch hour, and then eating when I got home from work until I went to sleep. It seemed to be my most happy time. I did not even realize that I was depressed at that time. My health got worse as each year went by. In 1998 I became disabled having diabetes, hypertension, sleep apnea, incontinence, morbid obesity and in a wheelchair.

In 2003 I made the best decision of my life. With God at my side, I decided to improve my health as by now I was having trouble breathing. I discussed stomach surgery with Dr. John Moon, III, my primary doctor. (I felt my days were numbered at this time in my life.) He told me I was making a good choice. So I researched the Internet to find a doctor that would do the laparoscopic gastric band surgery which would be less invasive. I found many and checked out the ones nearest to me. I made an appointment with Dr. Mark Watson, a surgeon at UT Southwestern about this procedure. He also agreed that I was making the right choice for me. He and his staff all treated me with kindness and understanding.

I scheduled my surgery for June 24, 2003, which was done at St. Paul Hospital. Twenty-seven months later I had lost 200 pounds. My health has very much improved. I no longer take insulin. My prescriptions went from thirteen down to five and those five are now a lower dosage. Best of all, no wheelchair.

How do I feel? Great!!! Now, I had some times that I would slip, for example, when I started back on solid food. I had this love affair with Cheetos. I talked with Michelle, the dietitian, and she was a big help to get me back on track. Then there was the time I bought one box, yes, just one box of Girl Scout Cookies® telling myself I would just eat two cookies each day. That night I ate all the cookies. I no longer buy Cheetos or Girl Scout cookies.

I joined a support group to help others who have had or are planning to have this stomach surgery. The Lord has now allowed me to help others also. My friends were there for me during the time of my weight loss. They provided me with clothes that fit as I lost my weight. I seemed to always have the size I needed. I found making a goal list is a very positive thing to do. I wanted to do things I could not do just 2 years ago and have accomplished many already. I have been horseback riding, rides on a Harley, dancing again, bowling, movies, concerts and the theater (now able to fit in the seats) and had a ride in an eighteen wheeler from Dallas to Houston and back.

I once got stuck in the seat at a hockey game at the Reunion Arena. After most people left, some gentlemen helped me get out. It was truly my most embarrassing moment. I can now go to sporting events with no concern. Other happy times... First time I could cross my legs, tie my shoes, put my socks on without help, pull up the car seat to get closer to the steering wheel, tuck in my blouse, wear jeans (no more elastic waist polyester pants) sit in a booth at a restaurant, and the list goes on.

I am currently a member of the Red Hat Society® and have made even more friends. I wrote a skit and performed in it with several other tiara tootin' tootsies at our 1 year anniversary celebration. I have been very active since my weight loss and have a lot of energy now with no breathing problems.

My social life now seemed to have only one thing missing. Yes, dating!!!!! I talked to my doctor about the feelings I was experiencing. Let's just say I was feeling very horny for the first time in the 13 years I went without a man in my life. I joined the American Legion Auxiliary in April 2004. That's where I met Geoffrey. He has made me feel young and alive. He is my best friend and I love him. He cares a lot about me and makes me laugh every day (among other things). Now it seems my calendar is so full that I have to schedule doctor appointments between activities in which I am involved.

If you are totally ready mentally to change your eating disorder then you can be successful too with this surgery. It is about focus one day at a time. (Where have we heard that before?) If I had to do it again? You bet I would. I had absolutely no problems with the surgery Dr. Watson performed. It has changed my life medically, physically, and mentally. I feel young again at age 65. (Geoffrey is 50 and "hot"!!!)

I am in the medical profession as a lab tech in a hospital. I decided to have weight loss surgery after much thought. I was tired. Just plain tired of trying and failing over and over again. My weight was affecting my personal and emotional life.

I have benefited from having the LAP-BAND in the way that it limits my portions, which was always a problem for me. It's the tool I need to say... 'stop.'

Anyone who is not looking for the 'fastest, quickest' weight loss would benefit from this surgery. I have lost 41 pounds in 8 months. I know that every pound lost is NOT coming back. It's gone for good. I have had no complications whatsoever. It has been a very smooth and positive experience and I would not hesitate for one second to do this again. I have no regrets whatsoever.

I did not take any meds for anything prior and really wasn't that active before LAP-BAND. Now I go to the gym every other day and can walk longer than I could before and don't get tired as quickly.

▼▼▼

I am a lecturer of law and an academic lawyer. My reason for having weight loss surgery was twofold. Firstly, I had exhausted all of the diet fads on the market. Secondly, the public relations and advertising for the surgery was quite persuasive.

The surgery has benefited me by teaching me to eat smaller portions.

The most suitable people for this surgery are those who are 300 pounds or heavier and those who are prepared to work with the program by exercising.

Frankly, I have not had any real problems with the surgery. It has been great to me. I have had the usual problems of regurgitation if I ate too quickly, but that is about all. I would have the operation all over again.

I had the surgery in January of 2005, and, to date, I have lost about 110 pounds.

After the surgery and once I began to drop pounds rapidly, I was removed from all medications—diabetes, high blood pressure, and apnea.

I am more active than I have been in 20 years. I am in the gym three times a week, walking, swimming, running—I do it all now.

▼▼▼

I am the broker/owner of a real estate office. I was 40 and 266 pounds, female and 5' 5". A business associate of mine had LAP-BAND, and I decided it was worth looking into. Secretly inside I was thinking that they would tell me that I wasn't a candidate, because I didn't see myself as a "fat" person. I went to the info sessions, and Dr. Jones was available for any questions. I can honestly say that he was a huge part of why I felt so comfortable making this decision. He has a way with people that I have never seen in a doctor.

After over 20 years of struggling with my weight, once I looked closer at my statistics and realized that I was truly a good candidate...I decided to have weight loss surgery. I had tried many, many programs and diets, and I was successful at losing weight, but not at keeping it off. Every 5 years I would gain back the 50 pounds that I had worked so hard to lose. I hit 40 years old, and I became more aware of the numerous heath problems that accompany people who are obese. I had joint problems, foot problems, borderline diabetes, and others.

The LAP-BAND works for me because I evaluated my bad eating patterns and realized that I would not eat all day and then eat a huge meal at dinner time, often full of carbs and fat. I wasn't eating during the day because I knew that I couldn't make a good food choice. I decided that it would be better not to eat than to eat the wrong food. Clearly this approach wasn't working, it wasn't healthy, and it was causing me to consume an entire day's calories at 7 p.m. The band works for me because now I can be in most any eating situation and unless I want to face an immediate negative consequence, I don't overeat. It takes a while to get used to that concept, but it works. You just say... enough is enough.

Now I eat breakfast, lunch and dinner and don't fear putting myself in eating situations because I know that I can eat small amounts and be done with it. For me, the fear of a blockage or extreme discomfort is enough to stop a feeding frenzy. Trust me, once you have your first experience with eating something too fast or without chewing enough... You feel like an elephant is standing on your chest and for the next 15 minutes you chant "I will never eat too fast again...just make the pain go away." Trust me, you think about it the next time.

I think that the LAP-BAND is best for eaters that have a problem with quantity eating. If you graze all day and eat small amounts of food, then this might not be for you. If you chew any type of food long enough, then you can eat it, and if you chewed all day, then you could consume large amounts of food. But if you are the type of person that eats very large portions of food and eats quickly when you do eat, then this certainly is a strong enough tool to deter that type of behavior.

I had no problems with the surgery or the Band, but I did have an allergic reaction to the tape that covered the incisions (with no previous history of allergies) and that turned into a fungal infection, which was very uncomfortable and not diagnosed properly for over 3 weeks. Keep the area dry!

I would definitely have the LAP-BAND again. The anxiety of the surgery was worse than the actual procedure. Don't be afraid when you can only consume six ounces of water 3 days after the surgery…your tolerance improves quickly, and in no time you will be drinking as they promise. I strongly encourage anyone considering the surgery to test the foods that you will be eating for the first few phases of the program before your surgery. You won't feel up to experimenting immediately after the surgery.

I had the surgery 3 1/2 months ago and have lost 40 pounds. I have had one fill. I find myself having much more energy, and since I am eating a more balanced diet, I really feel better than I ever have.

▼▼▼

I am a secretary who feels the LAP-BAND saved my life. I know I will live longer because of it. I enjoy life so much more because of the way I feel and look. My husband is a great support for me and very understanding when I vomit. I think it is very important to have people around you to support you. I am very lucky that my family is with me every step of the way. I do feel there should be more education to people considering the surgery. I don't think the physiologist I went to had enough information about the procedure. Dr. Jones and his staff are fantastic. I can't say enough about them. They do make this so much easier; they are there for me whenever I need them. I can't say enough good things about them. I feel they are my second family and I can talk to them about anything. I wish I could give them the gift they have given me, my life back. I had diabetes for 9 years before my surgery, and I just kept getting worse. My doctor at the Joslin Clinic (Dr. Hamdy), another lifesaver, introduced me to the program. I was taking four shots of insulin a day, anywhere from 125 to 150 units a day. Every day I felt like I was dying a little, and I haven't felt like that since my surgery. I am helping my older sister right now. She is considering the LAP-BAND.

I think anyone who is suffering with diabetes or is so overweight that it is affecting what they can and cannot do should consider having the procedure. If a person is considering LAP-BAND for a quick fix to lose weight, they should realize the life changes it is all about. I went to all the classes and to the physiologist, and I feel I still didn't realize what the surgery involved. I swelled up right after the surgery and I still don't know why I was in the hospital for 7 days after the surgery. I am still vomiting a lot and am uncomfortable. But I still feel it was worth it. My gall bladder was removed. I had the surgery 22 months ago and, to date, have lost 65 pounds. I am off of insulin and inhalers, and I can walk and talk at the same time and not lose my breath. I can do exercise and feel good.

In closing, I can't stress enough how much this LAP-BAND has helped me get a new life. I want to deeply express my appreciation to Dr. Jones and Angie and the rest of the staff for all their help and caring and support. Next to my husband, Dr. Jones is my hero.

▼▼▼

I have struggled with being overweight since childhood. I had only a brief period from age 15 to 19 that I weighed 120 pounds and didn't constantly have to worry about what I was consuming. After bearing three children within the following 4 years, I weighed an extra 50 pounds and felt very depressed about it. I had tried several diets and exercise routines only to lose 10 to 20 pounds, and then very quickly regain 30 plus pounds. I looked at photos of both my parents' families and could see obesity was a big problem on both sides. At 37 years of age and 240 pounds, I decided it was time to seek outside help and even go so far as to undergo surgery to regain control. I was tired of fighting a losing battle. I was beginning to have only a few of the problems associated with morbid obesity, acid reflux disease, low back pain, bilateral knee pain, and high cholesterol. I had started to take medications for some of these problems and knew more would be in my very near future if I didn't do something.

At that time, I was a registered nurse working in the PACU (Post-Anesthesia Care Unit—Recovery Room) in a very busy university hospital. Fortunately for me, our facility was (and still is) using state of the art technology and procedures to aid patients with various surgical procedures. It was in this arena that I learned of the LAP-BAND procedure. I took care of one of our first postoperative patients undergoing LAP-BAND at our facility. My curiosity got the best of me, and I began asking the surgeon questions about the Band and the procedure. I was told that there were informational meetings held at our facility. I attended a meeting to learn all that I could and have the opportunity to ask more questions of other surgeons providing this service. I must say I had quite an advantage. More so than any other person who was researching this new topic. I had access to patients who had undergone the procedure. I also worked in the pre-op area. This is the area where patients are prepped for surgery. I began seeing patients coming through pre-op who had LAP-BAND surgery 1 to 2 years prior and were coming back for cosmetic reconstruction. Not all were there for abdominoplasty. Many were there to have breast augmentation or liposuction. After speaking to all of these patients, each and every one said they would do it again and it was the best thing they could have done. I did not hear one negative comment from approximately 10 to 20 people that I questioned about their procedure. I asked how long they were off from work due to surgery and was quite surprised that many of them had the procedure on a Thursday and returned to work on Monday. They also said it was relatively easy to adjust their eating habits. Portion control was what I was looking for.

I contemplated for approximately 1 year before I made an appointment to see my surgeon. I was having anxiety issues with undergoing anesthesia—even though I worked with the doctors who would be putting me to sleep and trusted them wholeheartedly—I had never been anesthetized and quite frankly, it scared me. Once again, I was at an advantage. I was able to actually witness patients emerging from anesthesia, which ones could anticipate problems and which ones could be expected to do well. I finally overcame my fear and had my surgery December 19, 2005. To date, I have lost 68 pounds almost effortlessly.

For me the Band works just as I was told it would. My stomach is constricted to a point that only a small portion of food is able to enter. My surgeon and nursing staff warned me of what to expect if I ate too much, too fast. They were absolutely correct. The first 6 to 8 weeks after surgery one can expect to have liquids and advance to soft food until swelling decreases. During this time I was able to feel constriction. By the 7th to 8th week, the swelling had decreased, and I was able to consume more. I knew then it was time to have my first fill. The first 2 weeks after having the Band filled, I learned what happens to those who eat too much, too fast. Old habits began to resurface. Being a nurse, eating on the run is generally a must. I had to remind my brain that I had made a commitment. Otherwise I would have a negative response. For 2 weeks I had to remind myself, and generally it was after I had made myself sick and had food stuck in my food pipe. I must say that is a miserable feeling. But it still took me about 2 weeks for it to sink in—"You can no longer eat large quantities of food in a hurry!!!" I was able to go for several months without having another fill. By this time enough time had elapsed that once again I had to remind myself "Eat Slowly." I only had two to three episodes of spitting up after this fill. I realized at that time that old habits are never too far away and that this was still a learning experience. It was crucial that I continue to do what my physician told me to do—take small bites, chew thirty to forty times, eat slowly to allow time for the signal from the stomach to reach the brain, otherwise that last bite could send you over the edge; only eat the amount of the size of the palm of your hand (not including fingers); wait 2 hours after eating to drink. This is not to say that by this time I had not experienced some frustration. Approximately 1 to 2 weeks after my first two Band fills, I experienced tightening in my esophagus around my Band. This was always associated with taking the first bite of food. It felt like a spasm. The first time this happened I had already taken two to three bites of food. Needless to say, everything came back up. I don't think there is anything more frustrating than wanting to eat something that smells so good that you can literally taste it and then to have it come back up. I remember getting very angry when this happened. Fortunately, it only lasted for a few days until I made the conscious decision that I would take one bite, wait to see what happened and then proceed from there. I would have to take one bite, chew for two to three minutes and wait another two to three minutes to make sure it was going to go down. It is this process that allows me to enjoy the taste of food longer, and I fill up on less food this way. I can also eat almost anything that I want by using this method. As I said before, my problem was not necessarily quality of food but quantity. I still allow myself a sweet upon occasion. I am vigilant not to allow this to get out of hand, otherwise I have gone to all this trouble and expense only to sabotage myself. I like how I look and feel at this point, and I won't jeopardize that. I personally have had no complications from my surgery and don't anticipate any. I have stopped taking all pre-surgery meds and now only take my prescribed vitamins. Things that I do now that I didn't do before surgery include wearing some of my oldest daughter's clothes (she's 18). I have almost cleaned out all of my old clothes. I wear a swim suit in public without being so self-conscious. The people who are the best candidates for LAP-BAND surgery I think are those who will be committed not only to themselves but to trusting their doctor and doing what he says to do. Those who are not good candidates are those who refuse to open their minds to change. Change comes from within, and if someone is not ready or willing to make the necessary changes to take control of their situation, then there is no surgery or procedure out there that can fix the problem.

▼▼▼

I am a registered nurse who is the director of a home care company in suburban Boston, Massachusetts.

I had my surgery on March 14, 2006 after 45 plus years of struggling with weight issues. I tried everything from Weight Watchers (8 times) to OPTIFAST® to being admitted to an eating disorders unit (I left after 5 days) to having a staple placed in my ear to curb my appetite. Each time I had some positive results but not for long. After learning of the success rate of keeping the pounds off with the LAP-BAND procedure, I opted for this.

The benefit to me was that I was no longer hungry. I ate what was prescribed through the various stages post-op and NEVER EXPERIENCED HUNGER.

I have had a few minor instances of eating too fast or not chewing enough but those were a small price to pay for success. I have lost 48 pounds to date (5 months) but more importantly, 40 inches from my body (chest, waist, hips, calves and thighs). I can actually walk over two miles without dyspnea and can even climb stairs with no difficulty. I am off all three of my blood pressure medications, and my ankles hardly ever swell.

In addition to looking and feeling better physically, I feel better about myself. I feel like I have finally taken control over a lifelong problem, and my self-esteem has sky-rocketed. I even took a plane trip recently, something I had avoided since I had trouble fitting into the plane seats.

I think that the LAP-BAND is best for someone who is motivated and able to exercise daily. Without my daily treadmill routine of 30 to 40 minutes, I would not have been as successful.

▼▼▼

I decided to have weight loss surgery because I'm 42 years old, and I've tried so many diets and different ways to lose weight with no lasting results. I was able to lose weight with some of the diets but, I always put it back on plus more, each time getting more and more upset with myself. I needed help because I'd do well the first 3 weeks on any of the diets but then I'd plateau. That was okay for a week, sometimes 2 but then I'd get discouraged and end up eating the weight back on because I was so upset that the scale wouldn't budge. A friend of mine had gastric bypass but, to me that was just too drastic. I wanted to lose weight but the thought of re-routing my organs from their natural path and purposely malnutritioning my body to lose weight just wasn't for me. I often thought to myself, why can't they just do something to make you feel full sooner and make it last. One night, on the news they mentioned a new surgery that helped with weight loss that was less invasive and had less complications than gastric bypass, and they called it LAP-BAND® System. Right after the report, I got on the Internet and started researching. I knew right away that LAP-BAND was for me and finally felt relief that I would have help. I loved the fact that if something should happen, the band could be taken out and my organs would be back to normal. This was definitely the best decision I have made for myself. I'm not used to taking care of myself first but, THIS was something I knew I wanted for myself.

Benefits are not feeling that starving feeling between meals, being able to still have the foods I like but, in much better portions. It's helped me lose weight and keep it off. The band reminds me that I need to slow down my eating and to make better choices because the limited amount of food that fits in my stomach needs to be quality foods.

LAP-BAND keeps me from overeating, it helps me keep myself in check with my food choices yet, I don't feel deprived because I know if I really want something I can still have it. I felt from the beginning this was a tool to keep me on track and help me get past the plateaus before I blew it again. I'm not hungry in between meals like I used to be, therefore, I'm not eating the chocolate or other fatty snacks I used to. I now eat healthy portions instead of overdoing it. This tool has helped me in so many ways, and the benefit is I'm steadily losing weight and not feeling deprived or frustrated or that I'm out of control.

I think the person that is best for LAP-BAND is someone who realizes it's just a tool. This is not going to do all the work for you. This is definitely for someone who wants to feel in control of their weight loss because they truly are doing the work, but, this tool gives a hand in portion control. I don't think the Band is for the person who thinks this will make them popular or loved more. It's not for a person who's not going to take making the healthy food choices seriously and who's not going to do the aftercare. It's for the committed person, committed to doing better for him/herself for no one else but themselves. It's definitely not for someone who's losing weight for someone else.

I haven't had any complications. I have eaten too fast or didn't chew well enough and got that golf-ball feeling in my chest. I know that was my fault, and I learned from it. I would definitely have LAP-BAND again.

I had my surgery on February 13, 2006. I have lost 51 pounds so far (almost 6 months). I picture 5, 10 pound bags of potatoes and I just can't believe I used to carry that around. I'm looking forward to reaching my goal, but I'm being reasonable and make mini goals along the way. This will take time. Heck, it's taken me 42 years to put it on, so it should take some time to take it off.

I was on high blood pressure medication and came completely off of it for 3 months. Just this week my primary care physician put me on medication for high blood pressure again, but it's one-quarter the strength I used to be on. (Stress at my job I believe is causing this.) I'm able to go up flights of stairs and not be out of breath, I do much more yard work without getting tired, I feel so much more energy than before, and I've worn shorts for the first time in I don't know how many years.

I'm also able to get in and out of smaller bathroom stalls without hitting the sides of the walls/doors, my stomach no longer touches the car steering wheel, and when I get up in the morning I no longer have heel pain.

I am a medical billing supervisor for a company that does the billing for a very large physicians' organization. I supervise fourteen staff members, and we do billing for primary care physicians, psychiatry and radiation oncology. I'm also a wife (re-married a little over a year ago) and mother to a 16-year-old son.

▼▼▼

Three years, 85 pounds, and seven sizes ago, I decided to make a change in my life and had the LAP-BAND surgery. Obesity had always been a prominent feature in my family. Diabetes, high blood pressure, and knee and back pain were constant health conditions in most of my immediate and secondary family members. The year I turned 30, I made a decision that I did not want that to be my future anymore. I was tipping the scale at 225 on a 5' 1" frame, and my size 20 pants were starting to feel tighter. I knew that I could not fight the weight loss battle anymore, and I needed to contact someone who could help me change my perspective permanently towards eating and food.

I had always considered myself active because I was a retail manager and could "out walk" any of the younger kids who worked with me. However, over time, I was finding that going up ladders, lifting heavy boxes, and walking the sales floor were becoming increasingly more difficult, and those younger kids weren't lagging behind as much as they did in the past. I finally made a decision that enough was enough, and I contacted a surgeon who performed LAP-BAND surgery. Within a month of my initial consultation, I had the surgery and found myself on the road to a new life. I had no idea at the time how different that new life would be for me.

The first 3 months were probably the most difficult and challenging months in my life because I had to change 30 years of thinking and habits. I had to completely retrain myself on how to eat, what to eat, when to eat, and how much to eat. I went from eating half of a large pepperoni pizza to eating three bites and feeling full. Food that I used to love with a passion like rice, pizza, and pasta were no longer on the top of my taste buds' favorite list. I had to cut all carbonated drinks such as beer and soda out of my diet completely. I had to drastically limit the intake of foods I loved like ice cream, cakes, and cookies so that I didn't waste my meals on non-filling substances. Strangely, the most difficult part of my adjustment was getting used to the looks others gave when they saw the extremely small portions I consumed. At any given meal, I ate, at the most, 1/2 cup of food. But, trust me, that 1/2 cup made me feel full for the next 4 to 5 hours.

Initially, I had difficulty with my food portions and how to adjust my brain to my LAP-BAND. The LAP-BAND only allows a very small portion of food to enter your stomach every few hours. If I tried to eat even one bite more than what I should have, I would definitely know it within 2 minutes of that bite. I only had to "spit up" my food a few times before I learned the true meaning of portion control. I also had to train myself not to drink at least 1 hour before and 2 hours after eating. If I tried to work against this simple rule, I would find that I was famished within just a couple of hours of eating because I essentially washed all the food through my stomach.

My life has completely changed in the last 3 years. Those who knew me before my surgery do not even recognize the person I was 3 years ago. I've changed my perspective on exercise, food habits, and quality of life. I would say that I'm happier than I was before and not just because I am smaller. I honestly feel better about me. Four weeks after my surgery, I started walking and joined a gym. Now I run about three to five miles three times a week. I've done things that I've never done before like experiencing the great rush of excitement when you cross the finish line in a 5k race. I ran in an eight-mile race on Thanksgiving Day last year, which was definitely the highlight of my life. In the past, I would have been gorging from morning until night and taking afternoon naps on that day. But no more.

Currently, I weigh around 138 to 142 and wear a size 8 comfortably. I'm training for my second "Turkey Trot" race and hope to beat my last year's 90-minute time. I can't imagine my life without the LAP-BAND and would never go back. It's not a miracle, fix-it-all remedy for obesity. A person has to truly want to change her life to be successful with the LAP-BAND. It will make eating easier, but the individual person has to put in 98% of the work and dedication. I truly believe that anyone could be successful with the LAP-BAND. However, the motivation has to be more than just to be a smaller size. A person has to honestly want to be healthier and want to feel better about herself in order to make the LAP-BAND successful for her.

▼▼▼

I was beginning to have significant health problems, partially due to my weight. I had arthritis in my neck causing severe headaches and in my knees making it difficult to walk. I also experienced a great deal of difficulty sleeping and was starting to encounter symptoms of sleep apnea and snoring, much to my husband's dismay. I had tried all the usual diets, weight loss aids, and even been on a doctor-assisted weight loss program. Although I'd lose a few pounds here and there, they never stayed off and usually came back—with friends! I had a sit-down job working for a major telecommunications company at the time, so I got very little exercise at work. And even though our company had an exercise facility for its employees, I was uncomfortable working out in front of my coworkers and, frankly, I didn't have the energy or the stamina to even complete a minimal exercise program.

A coworker of mine had recently had the LAP-BAND surgery, and we began following her progress, which was dramatic. After watching her and talking with other people who had the surgery, I began investigating it for me. Finally, in May 2005, I had the surgery—the first surgery I'd ever had in my life.

After the surgery, I followed the doctor's orders carefully—which is the key to success of any program of this nature. The weight began dropping. Slowly, but very steadily. Ten pounds, then 20.. Soon I had to get some new clothes because my old ones were getting noticeably baggy. Within a year, I had dropped approximately 90 pounds and gone from a snug size 22 to a comfortable size 11/12 jeans, and a new lease on life. I was able to go on long walks with my husband for the first time since our son had been born, nearly 16 years before. I could exercise and not be too worn out to continue after 10 minutes. I went on my first 5k walk for a local fund-raising program and was not only able to complete the walk, but had energy left over afterwards!

The benefits of this surgery have been remarkable for me. Losing the weight was great! I now actually wear a size smaller than when I met my husband 24 years ago, I have more energy, my health has improved dramatically, and my husband is happy to inform me I don't snore anymore. But the improvement to my self-esteem and confidence level has been the biggest benefit. I feel much better about myself and look forward to doing things I was too insecure to do before. I see the pride in my husband's face when we greet friends we hadn't seen for a while. I take a more active role in my family's activities and was even confident enough to interview for and obtain a new job much closer to home with better benefits. I'm now a customer service manager for a large company, providing support for the entire East coast—something I would never have had the confidence to do before.

I've been very happy with my decision to have this surgery and would recommend it for anyone significantly overweight who is willing to follow the doctor's directions and put in a little effort. It does require a change in lifestyle – small for me, more drastic for others. I try to eat healthier and stay active now, but

I find it so much easier that it never seems like the burden it did before my surgery. I've never had any complications nor inconveniences from the LAP-BAND. Even now, 16 months after my surgery, I'm not gaining weight back, nor do I feel deprived in any way. I am happier and healthier than I've been in nearly 20 years and love it when people call me "Slim" or say that I don't look anywhere close to the 45 I'll turn in a couple weeks!

▼▼▼

I had the LAP-BAND procedure in December of 2004. I had been overweight a majority of my life. I remember being the chubby one throughout my years in school. I continued to gain weight through college and even after college. I tried numerous diets, and nothing seemed to work. At the age of 24, I had basically determined I would always be obese. At the same time, several of my family members started having health problems from being overweight. One of my relatives called me one day and asked me to go with her to an informational meeting about weight loss surgery. I went to be supportive with absolutely no intention of having any type of surgery myself. The thought of surgery seemed drastic and scary. At the meeting, however, I liked what I heard. The Lap-Band procedure seemed like a great option for someone my age for several reasons. First of all, it is reversible if something ever goes wrong. Second, it is adjustable to accommodate the changes of my weight throughout my life. Third, there would be little recovery time. I still left the meeting not so convinced it was the right thing for me.

My family member who I went to the meeting with decided to have the surgery. Over the next few months, I watched her progress and was amazed. One day, I suddenly realized that I wanted to have the LAP-BAND surgery. Once I made the decision, there was no turning back. Three months later, I had the surgery. At this point, I was determined to lose weight. I followed the diet plan and was very careful of the types of food I ate. I really focused on getting lots of protein and a few vegetables. The best and easiest food I found to eat was grilled fish. Along with the diet, I started a workout routine. I started out slow and eventually built up to 30 to 45 minutes a day on the elliptical machine. I continued this until I met my weight loss goal. Approximately 14 months after my surgery date, I had lost 130 pounds! I had gone from 280 pounds to 150 pounds! I lost a whole person! The best part was that I met my goal just in time to order my wedding dress. Two years earlier as a size 24, I never would have dreamed that I would be getting married in a size 8 wedding dress! The wedding was only a couple of months ago, and I'm still glowing from the day. I felt like the most beautiful bride. I really had come a long way.

There are a few things that I have learned from my experience as well as others in my support group. Most importantly, you should only have this surgery if you are committed to put forth some effort. The LAP-BAND is only a tool, not a solution. That was the best advice Dr. Watson gave me. You still must watch what you eat and stay away from high fat food as much as possible. Remember, it is possible to have this surgery and still gain weight. However, don't deprive yourself of something you are really craving, just indulge in a treat occasionally. The second thing I have learned is that you must focus on eating protein combined with a steady workout routine. It doesn't have to be heavy workouts, just consistent. Lastly, you must surround yourself with supportive family and friends. Support groups are vital to success. It's important to share experiences with other people going through the same thing, to know you aren't alone and to know that when you do have a little stumble, you can pick yourself right back up and continue on just like everyone else.

I am proud that I had the surgery and the success that I've had with it. I am a new and improved person both physically and emotionally. I hope that my story helps others make the right decision for their lives.

▼▼▼

As I celebrate my third 'Second Birthday', (I consider it my 'second birthday' because that is the day I received a 'new life)

I cannot help but reflect upon the numerous beneficial changes which have occurred during these past three years. I achieved every one of my original goals – no insulin, no medications and getting rid of the extra 100 lbs from this body. Last year, I was shocked by being 'kicked out of' the diabetes clinic. My A1C was too low to qualify as their patient!! To quote The Great One, "How sweet it is!" – pun intended. Moreover, I discovered that my uterine fibroids have disappeared along with their symptoms! Subsequently, I no longer have to worry about the excess fat's generating extra estrogen causing any harm – namely cancer. I, along with my other doctors, never saw that one coming. I consider it a real plus to my continued good health. Thanks to these changes, I will live to be a healthy 103!

But these are just the medical benefits. Important? Definitely! However, they are not the only benefits. Just recently someone sent me a photo of myself taken approximately three months before the procedure. I could not believe the drastic change. No wonder my cousin did not recognize me at his daughter's wedding. (He did when I swore at him in Italian.J) When I saw that photo, my life at that time came back and the many changes since flooded me with a joy I can only hope others have experienced.

I can shop in a regular store and not dread the experience. I can even find exceptional sale prices in my size. For someone who has paid close to $200 for a bathing suit because it existed and FIT, nothing compares to the feeling of NOT having to settle. Also, I can fit in a regular train seat and not stand the whole time because of the rude comments from other riders. I no longer need an extension on a flight and even have 12" of extra strap now with the armrests around me. The significant increase in my energy level is phenomenal. Although, I have always been active – I do not tire as easily. Moreover, people actually acknowledge me when I approach a service counter – a far cry from the 'looking past you' experiences of the past. I can even order an ice cream and NOT have a complete stranger take it away, while telling you, "Stop eating. You need to go on a diet." while other patrons laughed. (In case you were wondering, it takes 4 seconds for the brain to register what is said, for you to get up off your seat and go after the person. The manager got to him first. Twenty-five years later I am still waiting for this guy's return. That day will prove to be interesting on Cape Cod. J)

As a Christmas gift, my nieces gave me acrobat lessons! When I arrived, I noticed a weight limit and was happy to see I was well under the maximum limit. What a delight! I took the lessons and was soaring through the air after about 4 hours. I never would have been able to do so at my old weight. I also learned how to trail ride this summer and did not feel badly for the horse given my new weight. I actually got her to trot – what an experience for this urban animal lover. I went dog sledding in Canada last year – what a thrill! My next goals are sky diving and pilot lessons. Weight limits are no longer an issue. I am living a 'normal' life.

These are a mere smattering of benefits. There are countless other incidents for which I will be eternally grateful. However, that is a book in itself. It is the simple everyday things 'normal weighted' people take for granted which have the most memorable impact. I will never take them for granted, since I cherish each and every one of them.

The crowning moment came the day of my revision. I had prayed either for a band or Roux – en Y. If not, then I prayed God would take me. Living my old lifestyle is not an option – period. When I awoke and felt the port – 'A Second Chance!.' My gratitude and joy cannot be put into words. I do not and will not take this band for granted: I will do whatever is necessary to keep it functioning properly – period.

Concluding, thanks to your sharp mind, caring heart and skillful hands, I have and will be fulfilling many of my childhood dreams. "THANK YOU!" is just not enough. When you have those days when things are not 'nice', remember I am only one of many whom you have helped live the 'normal life'. The others may not have verbalized their gratitude; I can assure you every one of them is grateful for all that you have done. All the best!

▼▼▼

My decision for weight-loss surgery was more than a year in thought and discussion with my family. The good news, my husband was supportive, the bad news, now that I made the statement, what was I going to do about it? Just prior to my vacation last summer I was sick and tired of being sick and tired...my joints and back hurt, I had multiple co-morbidities and was afraid of having "frequent flyer miles" at the pharmacy.

When I finally realized that my health issues were probably directly connected to my weight I was ready. It was time to get serious. With about 100 lbs. to lose, I decided the lap-band was the tool that would allow me to be totally invested in my own weight-loss progress.

- I have had no complications, only (2) fills = 1.5cc total with excellent restriction and satiety.

- I often speak at information sessions in our area and tell new patients both the band and gastric bypass are weight-loss tools, and both can achieve excellent results BUT the individual has to "be sick and tired of being sick and tired." In other words, if they aren't ready to do the work, and be totally committed to changing their current behaviors, then the success they achieve is only temporary. A positive attitude, new behaviors, commitment to exercise, follow-up appointments, and communication are the key to winning this game – the patient is the captain of the team, and the WLS program, the coaches cheering the patient toward each success.

The metamorphosis for me has been outstanding. I am now walking pain-free at least 5 miles/day, walking up and down many flights of stairs without respiratory difficulty, all medications have been discontinued, and I sleep better. I'm enjoying the compliments regarding new image and people who know me say I look 10 years younger!

It has been a little over a year; I have lost 70 pounds and a total of 20.65 inches.

As an RN, I know the incidence of obesity and age-related illness. I'm happy to have a tool to help me be proactive in my healthy weight management plan. This is the best birthday present I could have ever bought myself!! (surgery was the day after my BD) Life is good; I am over 50 and fabulous!

GREAT TOOL – I'd do it again, but sooner this time!

Tell your story.
Log on to
www.lapbandcompanion.com
and share your struggles and successes.
Post "before" and "after" photo
and track weight loss.

▼▼▼
New Health

Weight-loss surgery utilizing the LAP-BAND is not just a program to allow you to arrive at a particular new weight. It is not just to have the world no longer see you as a heavy person. The real goal is to emerge and enter the world with your new-found health. It may be impossible to predict the improvement in your life because many things you deal with on a daily basis are related to weight, and you do not realize it. Of course, other drudgeries are unrelated to weight.

Imagine being able to participate in physical activities that are difficult for you that many others always take for granted. As a simple example, walking or even running for more than short distances by having not only the ability, but also the energy and desire to do it. For some, this can be as miraculous as throwing away canes and crutches and getting up out of wheelchairs. For others, it can allow a simple stroll in the park or through the mall with family or friends—this time, however, without gasping for air or having pain in the legs or back.

Simply taking a pill or completing a short course of therapy will not accomplish this goal. It will require your starting a journey that will require your attention and involvement. This journey will not be taken alone however; you will be part of a larger team. At times, it may not be easy. It is not a "one-stop shop." But you can do it. Many others before you have. The intense participation on your part can produce a deep sense of accomplishment in your heart.

Think about your personal health issues at the present time. Think about the medications, therapies, and/or equipment that are needed throughout the day to keep you going. Envision leaving this stuff behind. Consider the simplicity and economy. Medications for diabetes or high blood pressure could be reduced or eliminated and become part of your past. The need for CPAP to keep you breathing at night could go into the closet as sleep apnea resolves.

At the same time, you might bring other things out of the closet. Clothes you wore in the past could start to fit and also might come back into style. Sports equipment you thought you could never use again might become part of your new routine.

For others, losing weight with the Band could mean being able to have a new child, and the health and energy to care for the child. Some people struggle with their specialists to find a treatment for their infertility. Many times, a reduction in weight is the key to ending menstrual irregularities and improving fertility. Once pregnant, women are much better prepared to carry the additional weight of the child growing inside of them. Once you deliver, chasing the child through the house or park is much easier.

The examples are too numerous to cover.

You must weigh the risks and benefits of surgery. You must ask yourself, "Am I ready for a lifestyle change, healthy diet and regular exercise?"

It is our wish that the information in this book will assist you, as it has the hundreds in our practice, to achieve your new health.

Mark J. Watson, M.D.

Daniel B. Jones, M.D.

Appendices

Appendix 1

Online Resources

For more information, visit:

www.lapbandcompanion.com

www.Bandsters.net

www.ASMBS.org

www.SAGES.org

www.obesityaction.org

www.lapbandtalk.com

www.band2gether.com

www.thebostonchannel.com

www.bariatricedge.com

www.lapband.com

www.obesityeducation.com

www.obesityhelp.com

www.BIDMC.harvard.edu/wls

www.utsouthwestern.edu

Appendix 2

Reflections From a Weight-Loss Surgery Support Group

Before Surgery...

I'd be sitting there in my doctor's office, 200 pounds overweight, and he wouldn't even ask about it!

Doctors would say to me, "Oh, you're overweight...you must be depressed...here's some Prozac."

Obesity is a sickness, a disease. Just like anorexia.

When I decided to have my surgery, I had hit rock bottom. It was like being an alcoholic. I just HAD to do something drastic—I couldn't go on the way I was.

Being fat—what did I hear all the time? "You must be lazy...you must be sloppy...ah you have such a pretty face."

It's like people saw an inverse relationship between how big my butt was and how small my brain must be.

Isn't it nice to have any option? (with reference to having surgery to consider)

After Surgery...

Getting surgery isn't the easy way out. Many people made value judgments about my choice—"Couldn't you just have dieted and done it yourself?" But getting this procedure was a huge life change, from changing what I eat to my entire social situation.

The whole procedure is the greatest thing in the world. Now I jump out of bed to get onto a scale, and I feel like I am going to be born again.

A common fear among patients who have had the surgery—"I'm afraid to start eating solids again—I am scared of putting on weight, afraid it will start all over again."

Getting surgery was NOT the easy way out. But it changed my whole life. The surgery itself was really only a small part of it.

I consider my surgery day my birthday—I started over then.

Appendix 3
Meal Meter (Food Log)

Food Item During the Meal (Time _____)

_____
Food Item (Solid Protein)

_____
Amount (Bites, Tbs, Cups)

Consistency: ☐ Solid   ☐ Soft   ☐ Liquid

Food Item During the Meal (Time _____)

_____
Food Item (Solid Protein)

_____
Amount (Bites, Tbs, Cups)

Consistency: ☐ Solid   ☐ Soft   ☐ Liquid

Food Item During the Meal (Time _____)

_____
Food Item (Solid Protein)

_____
Amount (Bites, Tbs, Cups)

Consistency: ☐ Solid   ☐ Soft   ☐ Liquid

Liquids During Meal

☐ **None**

Type _____

Amount _____

Calories _____

Result ──────────────▶ Changes

☐ Satisfied

☐ No change needed
working well

_____

☐ Spit-up

☐ Decrease amount next meal
    ☐ Number of Bites _____

☐ Heartburn

    ☐ Size of Bites
    ☐ Total Amount_____

☐ Pain

☐ Call bariatric office if no improvement
with change

_____

☐ Not full or satisfied

☐ Stop drinking with meal or before/after
☐ More solid food consistency
☐ Call bariatric office if no improvement
(Dietitian adjustment)

Time When I Began Drinking After Meal

_____

Time When I Was Hungry Again

_____

Snack?   **☐ None**

Yes _____
    Food/Calories

Appendix 4

Clinical Pathways

	Before Your Surgery	Day of Surgery	Day After Surgery
What to do today	☐ You may NOT eat after midnight before your surgery	☐ You will not be able to eat ☐ You may walk short distances with assist at least once, more if tolerated ☐ You may perform breathing exercises 10 times/hour while awake ☐ Wear your compression boots when not ambulating to prevent blood clots in your legs	☐ You will have a swallow study ☐ You may begin a Stage I diet and progress to Stage III diet if you pass your swallow study ☐ You may sit edge of bed for all meals ☐ You may walk independently ☐ You may perform breathing exercises 10 times/hour while awake ☐ Wear your compression boots when not ambulating to prevent blood clots in your legs
Activity	• Continue with your normal daily exercise routine 30 minutes daily	• You may sit edge of bed	• You should walk in the hall by yourself at least three times
Education	• Review the handout on pre-op dietary restrictions	• You will learn how to use the pain scale • You will learn how to perform breathing exercises	• An inpatient nurse practitioner will review the patient education packet and support group information

	Before Your Surgery	Day of Surgery	Day After Surgery
Tests/Procedures	• Your appointment with pre-aadmission test center is complete • Please use your Hibiclens or PhisoHex wash as per instructions from the nurse in the pre-admission test center	• The tube in your bladder may be removed • Your incision dressing will stay on • You may have your blood sugar checked	• Your incision dressing will be changed • You may have your blood sugar checked • You may have a blood test
Medications	• Please discontinue use of aspirin 10 days prior to surgery	• You may have IV pain medications	• You may have oral pain medications

Your Name: _____ Date of Surgery: _____

Surgeon Name: _____ Case Manager: _____

Home Discharge Criteria	Patient Discharge Information

☐ You can be discharged home when:
☐ Your vital signs (blood pressure, heart rate, etc.) are stable
☐ You can walk safely and at your activity level prior to surgery
☐ You are tolerating a Stage III diet
☐ You can urinate on your own
☐ Your pain scale is 1–4 on oral pain medication
☐ You and/or your family understand your medications
☐ Your wound care can be performed at home by you, your family, or a visiting nurse
☐ You and/or your family understand your diet instructions
	☐ You should understand the instructions for your discharge
	☐ Prescriptions are given for medications to go home
	Follow-up Bariatric appointment:
	Place:_____ _____/_____
	                    Date Time
	Next support group meeting:
	Place:_____ _____/_____
	                    Date Time
	When you are home, if you have any medical concerns, please call the Bariatric Clinic
	If you have any nutrition questions, please call the Nutrition Clinic

Appendix 5
Definition of Terms

ACS – American College of Surgeons

AP BAND – Cushioned band

ASMBS – American Society for Metabolic and Bariatric Surgery

Band – The part of the appliance that tightens around the stomach

BMI – Body mass index

Calorie – Measure of energy

Dumping – Passing food too quickly

Erosion – Wearing away of tissue by pressure of Band

Esophagus – Throat and food pipe

Esophageal Dilation – Stretching esophagus

Fluoroscopy – X-ray for looking at Band position

Gastrografin – Contrast agent for X-ray examinations

% EWL – Percent excess weight loss (extra weight above ideal)

Perforation – Hole in tissue

Perigastric – Around the stomach

Port – The hub of Band that is under the skin

Prolapse – Herniation of bottom of stomach through Band

Saline – Sterile water

VG Band – Largest band

Appendix 6
Your Before and After
Picture Journal

Before Surgery

Three Months After Surgery

Six Months After Surgery

Twelve Months After Surgery

18 months After Surgery

24 months After Surgery

Find a Surgeon in Your Area

Alabama

Jeffrey Caylor, DO

Tim Christopher, MD
Cahaba Valley Surgical
Group, PC

Ronald Clements, MD
University of Alabama

Kevin Cottingham, MD

Andrew DeWitt, MD
Caraway Physicians
Plaza III

Edward Facundus, MD

Kenneth Foreman, MD
Alabama Surgical
Associates, P.C.

Jeffrey Hannon, MD

Daniel Lane, MD
Surgical Associates of
Mobile

Ravindra Mailapur, MD
The Bariatric Center at
Huntsville Hospital

John Mathews, MD
The Surgeons
Group, P.C.

Robert Miles, MD

W. Pennington, MD

Forrest Ringold, MD

Lee Schmitt, MD

Ronald Smith, MD

William Suggs, MD
Surgery Consultants of
Decatur

John Touliatos, MD

Jefferson Vaughan, MD

L. Weinstein, MD

Arkansas

John Baker, MD

Mark Gibbs, MD

K. Bruce Jones, MD
NEA Clinic

Rex Luttrell, MD
Luttrell Surgical
Associates

William McAlexander, MD

J. Wellborn, Jr., MD

Arizona

Andrew Aldridge, MD
Flagstaff Surgical
Associates

Robert Berger, MD
Flagstaff Surgical
Associates

Robin Blackstone, MD
Scottsdale Bariatric
Center, PLC

Stephen Burpee, MD

Patrick Chiasson, MD

Daniel Fang, MD

David C. Johnson, MD
Salt River Bariatrics

Hilario Juarez, MD

Jennefer Kieran, MD

Amy Koler, MD
Scottsdale Bariatrics

Christopher Salvino, MD,
MS, MT

Rob Schuster, MD
Dept. of MIS-Stanford

Steven Simon, MD

Terry Simpson, MD
Arizona Bariatric Center

Alexander Villares, MD

California

Alberto Aceves, MD

Mir Ali, MD

Horacio Asbun, MD

Aaron Baggs, MD
Kaiser Permanente
Medical Center

Gary Belzberg, MD

Bobby Bhasker-Rao, MD
Advanced Laparoscopic &

Bariatric Surgery

Helmuth Billy, MD

Mathew Brunson, MD

Charles Callery, MD

Guilherme Campos, MD
University of California,
San Francisco

Philip Chin, MD

Paul Cirangle, MD

Sheilah Clayton, MD

Antonio Coirin, MD

John Coon, MD

Scott Cunneen, MD
Cedars-Sinai Med.
Center

Shyam Dahiya, MD

Parviz Daniels, MD

David Davtyan, MD
Beverly Hills Weight
Loss, Medical Clinic

David Deutsch, MD

Phillip Dickinson, MD

Francisco Espinosa-
Torres, MD

Mary Estakhri, MD

Edward Felix, MD

John Feng, MD
Crystal Springs Surgical
Associates, A Medical
Group, Inc.

David Fisher, MD
Kaiser Permanente

Pamela Foster, MD

Kelly Francis, MD

John Garcia, MD

Carlos Gracia, MD

Eric Hahn, MD
The Permanente Medical
Group, Inc.

Andrew Hajduczek, MD
Coastal Center for
Obesity

Sami Hamamji, MD

Ziad Hanna, MD, DO

Renetta Hatcher, MD

Kelvin Higa, MD
Advanced Laparoscopic
Surgery Associates

John Husted, MD
Pacific Laparoscopy

Daniel Igwe, Jr., MD

Hormuz Irani, MD

Elaine James, MD

Gregg Jossart, MD
California Pacific Medical
Center

Namir Katkhouda, MD
USC Dept. of Surgery

Ara Keshishian, MD
Central Valley Bariatrics

Theodore Khalili, MD

Stanley Klein, MD
Harbor - UCLA Medical
Center

Jeremy Korman, MD

Aaryan Koura, MD

Douglas Krahn, MD
Western Bariatric, AMC

Pedro Kuri, MD

Ariel Ortiz Lagardere, MD

Yen-Chung Lee, MD

Peter LePort, MD

Robert Li, MD
Kaiser South
San Francisco

Carson Liu, MD

Matthew Lublin, MD

Andrew Luckey, MD

Deron Ludwig, MD
General and
Bariatric Surgery

Laura Machado, MD
Sacramento Bariatric
Medical Associates

Arash Mahdavi, DO

Daniel Marcus, MD

Eufrocino Martinez, MD
New Reflections

Stephen McColgan, MD

Robert McKeen, MD
Southbay Bariatrics

Carie McVay, MD

Martha Morales, MD

John Morton, MD
Stanford School of
Medicine

George Mueller, MD
San Diego Bariatric
Surgeons

Nirav Naik, MD
Bakersfield Surgical
Associates

H. Naim, MD
Advanced Bariatric
Center

Dat Nguyen, MD

Ninh Nguyen, MD
University of CA, Irvine
Medical Center

David Oliak, MD

Fernando Otero, MD

Milton Owens, MD
Coastal Center for
Obesity

Judith Park, MD

Steven Patching, MD
Sutter Medical Center

Mahbod Paya, MD

Edward Phillips, MD

Alessio Pigazzi, MD
City of Hope

Andrew Posselt, MD, PhD
University of California,
San Francisco

Brian Quebbemann, MD
The New Program

Philippe Quilici, MD

John Rabkin, MD

Robert Rabkin, MD
Pacific Laparoscopy

Stanley Rogers, MD

Barry Sanchez, MD
Peninsula Surgical
Specialists Med. Group

Michelle Savu, MD
VA San Diego Healthcare
Center

Daniel Swartz, MD
Advanced Bariatric
Centers of California

David Thoman, MD

Ajay Upadhyay, MD

Don Van Boerum, MD

Donald Waldrep, MD

L. Wetter, MD

John Yadegar, MD

Karim Zahriya, MD

Colorado

John Bealer, MD

Reginald Bell, MD

Timothy Brown, MD

Frank Chae, MD
National Bariatric Center

Doru Georgescu, MD

Michael Johnell, MD
North Colorado
Medical Center

Gerald Kirshenbaum, MD

Robert Quaid, MD
Northern Colorado
Surg. Assoc., PC

Moses Shieh, DO

James Smith, MD

Michael Snyder, MD

Richard Tillquist, MD
Colorado Bariatric
Surgery/ SurgOne, P.C.

Connecticut

Jonathan Aranow, MD
Shoreline Surgical
Associates

Denise Barajas, MD

Carlos Barba, MD

Robert Bell, MD
Yale University

Laura Choi, MD

Timothy Ehrlich, MD
Fairfield County Bariatrics
& Surgical Spec.

Scott Ellner, DO
Saint Francis Hospital

Craig Floch, MD
Fairfield County Bariatrics
& Surgical Spec.

Neil Floch, MD
Fairfield County Bariatrics
& Surgical Spec.

Jeannine Giovanni, MD

Bruce Molinelli, MD
Surgical Specialists of
Greenwich

Geoffrey Nadzam, MD

Athanassios Petrotos, MD

Abdel Richi, MD

Oluseun Sowemimo, MD
Hospital of Saint Raphael

Darren Tishler, MD

Elmer Valin, MD

District of Columbia

Paul Lin, MD
George Washington
Hospital

Brian Long, MD
Foxhall Surgical
Associates, PC

Delaware

Isaias Irgau, MD

Michael Peters, MD

Gail Wynn, MD

Florida

Robert Bailey, MD

Thomas Bass, MD

Wiljon Beltre, MD

Glenn Burleson, MD

Patricia Byers, MD

Juan Cabrera, MD
Surgical Weight
Loss Institute

Carlos Carrasquilla, MD

Brett Cohen, MD

Robert Cywes, MD, PhD
Jacksonville Surgical
Associates

Nestor de la Cruz-Munoz, MD

David Diaz, MD
Mount Sinai Medical
Center

Richard DiCicco, MD
Florida Obesity Surgical
Associates

John Dietrick, MD

Rodolfo Dy, MD

Jose Erbella, Jr., MD

Paul Esposito, MD

Jose Estigarribia, MD

Juan-Carlos Fleites, MD

Mark Fusco, MD

Scott Gallagher, MD
Tampa General Hospital

Eddie Gomez, MD

Lee Grossbard, MD
Pasco Surgical
Associates

Barry Haicken, MD

Timothy Hipp, MD
Surgical Group of
Gainesville

Tiffany Jessee, DO
SunCoast Surgical
Specialists

Muhammad Jawad, MD
Bariatric & Laparoscopy
Center

Pachavit Kasemsap, MD

Keith Kim, MD

Pandurangan Krishnaraj, MD

Kenneth Larson, MD

Mark Liberman, MD
Cleveland Clinic Florida

Jeffrey Lord, MD
Sacred Heart Institute for
Surgical Weight Loss

Karen MacKenzie, MD
Surgical Obesity
Solutions

Robert Marema, MD

Ronald Moore, Jr., MD
Minimally Invasive
Surgery Inc.

Michel Murr, MD
Tampa General Hospital

William Overcash, MD

Michael Perez, MD
U.S. Bariatric

Mallik Piduru, MD

Ernest Rehnke, MD

Raul Rosenthal, MD
Cleveland Clinic of FL

Joel Sebastien, MD

Theodore Small, MD
Surgical Associates of
West Florida

C. Smith, MD
Mayo Clinic - Jacksonville

Scott Stevens, MD
Intercoastal Surgical
Group

Samuel Szomstein, MD
Cleveland Clinic Florida

Eric Valladares, MD
South Florida Surgery /
Bariatrics Institute

Arthur Verga, MD

G. Webb, MD
North Florida
Surgeons, P.A.

A. Whittwell, MD

Paul Wizman, MD

Natan Zundel, MD

Georgia

John Angstadt, MD

D. Ash, MD
Commerce Surgical
Assoc.

Vito Bagnato, MD
Albany Surgical

Michael Blaney, MD
Jones, Engler, Hill and
Blaney

Joseph Burnette, MD

J. Champion, MD

Ijeoma Ejeh, MD

Charles Finley, MD

Richard Fromm, MD
Dalton Surgical Group

Christopher Hart, MD

Peter Henderson, MD
Georgia Coast
Surgical, LLC

John Hunter, MD
Cedar Surgical
Associates, PC

William Johnson, MD

Harold Kent, MD
Georgia Coast
Surgical, LLC

Leena Khaitan, MD
Emory University Hospital

Edward Lin, DO
Emory University Hospital

Paul Macik, MD

John McKernan, MD, PhD
Center for Videoscopic
and Laser Surgery, Inc.

Sergio Mejias, MD

Steven Paynter, MD

Jaime Ponce, MD
Dalton Surgical
Group, PC

C. Procter, MD
Surgical Specialist of
Georgia

Robert Richard, MD

J. Ryland Scott, MD
Harbin Clinic

Dennis Smith, Jr., MD
Advanced Obesity
Surgery, LLC

Scott Steinberg, MD

Oliver Whipple, MD
Savannah Colon & Rectal
Surgery

Michael Williams, MD

Mark Wulkan, MD

Hawaii

Steven Fowler, MD
ALOHA Surgery, LLC

Brandt Lapschies, MD
Hawaii Bariatric Surgery
Center, Inc.

Kenric Murayama, MD
John A. Burns School of
Medicine, University of
Hawaii

Carlos Weber, MD
Kaiser Moanalua Medical
Center

Iowa

Thom Lobe, MD
Blank Children's Hospital

Denville Myrie, MD
Myrie Surgical
Associates, PC

Idaho

Eric Baird, MD

Robert Cahn, MD

David Chamberlain, DO
Chamberlain General
Surgery

Brian O'Byrne, MD

John Pennings, MD
Surgical Bariatrics
Northwest

Illinois

Andrew Agos, MD

Subhashini Ayloo, MD

Kathryn Bass, MD

Steven Bonomo, MD

Gerald Cahill, MD

James DeBord, MD

Bruce Dillon, MD

Constantine Frantzides,
MD, PhD
Chicago Institute of
Minimally Invasive
Surgery

Reza Gamagami, MD

Paul Guske, MD
Arlington Lakes
Professional Center

Amir Heydari, MD

Daniel Hoeltgen, MD

Eric Hungness, MD
The University of Chicago
Medical Center

Michael Iwanicki, DO

Christopher Joyce, MD
BMI Surgery

Mark Kadowaki, MD

David Klem, MD
DuPage Surgical
Consultants, Ltd.

Brian Lahmann, MD
Midwest Comprehensive
Bariatrics

Rami Lutfi, MD
Chicago Bariatric Institute

James Madura, II, MD
Rush University Medical
Center

Roger Maillefer, MD

J. Marshall, MD

Leslie McClellan, MD
Mercy Bariatric Wellness
Center

Alex Nagle, MD

Vivek Prachand, MD
University of Chicago,
Dept. of Surgery

Jay Prystowsky, MD
Northwestern Univ.
Medical School

Peter Rantis, Jr., MD
Arlington Lakes
Professional Center

Anthony Raspanti, MD

Sidney Rohrscheib, MD
Illinois Bariatric Center

Thomas Rossi, MD

Vafa Shayani, MD
Loyola University Medical
Center

Jonathan Spitz, MD

John Sutyak, MD
Southern Illinois Univ.
School of Medicine

Frederick Tiesenga, MD

Duane Tull, MD

Jonathan Wallace, MD

William Watson, MD

Indiana

Rafael Azuaje, MD

Brenda Cacucci, MD

Steven Clark, MD
Premier Surgical

John Ditslear, III, MD

Christopher Evanson, MD

Winston Gerig, MD

Gerardo Gomez, MD
IU-Wishard Trauma
Center

Christine Gupta, MD

Christopher Haughn, MD
Evansville Surgical

Steven Hoekstra, MD

RoseMarie Jones, MD
Carmel Surgical
Specialists

Samer Mattar, MD

Keith McEwen, MD

Denise Murphy, MD

Gregory Pulawski, MD

James Ray, MD

Don Selzer, MD

Mark Shina, MD

Dale Sloan, MD
St. Joseph Hospital

Paul Stanish, MD

Charles Stone, MD
Team Bariatric Center for
Weight Reduction

Kansas

Bernita Berntsen, MD
Tallgrass General &
Vascular Surgery

Carlyle Dunshee, II, MD

James Hamilton, Jr., MD

C. Hitchcock, MD
The Bariatric Center of
Kansas City

Stanley Hoehn, MD
The Bariatric Center of
Kansas City

Wanda Kaniewski, MD
The Institute for
Advanced Bariatric
Surgery

Brent Lancaster, MD

Paramjeet Sabharwal, MD
The Institute for
Advanced Bariatric
Surgery

Niazy Selim, MD

Brent Steward, MD
Tallgrass General Surgery

Abdel Tayiem, MD

Kentucky

Jeff Allen, MD
University of Louisville

Alex Argotte, MD

Edwin Gaar, MD
VA Medical Center

Vincent Lusco, III, MD
Louisville Surgical
Associates

John Oldham, Jr., MD
Bluegrass Bariatric
Surgical Associates,
PLLC

John Olsofka, MD
Louisville Surgical
Associates

Jorge Rodriguez, MD
University of Louisville

Dwayne Smith, MD
Advanced Bariatric
Centers, PLLC

Tom Sonnanstine, MD

Joshua Steiner, MD

Roderick Tompkins, Jr.,
MD

Laura Velcu, MD

G. Weiss, MD
Bluegrass Bariatric
Surgical Associates

Timothy Wheeler, MD
Surgical Weight Loss
Center

Louisiana

James Barnes, MD

Stephanie Barnes, MD

Drake Bellanger, MD
Advanced Videoscopic
Surgery of Baton Rouge

Keith Chung, MD

Andrew Hargroder, MD

Mark Hausmann, MD
Surgical Specialty Group

Colleen Kennedy, MD
Ochsner Clinic
Foundation

Teresa Klainer, MD

Thomas Lavin, MD

Karl Leblanc, MD, MBA

Wagih Mando, MD

Christa Mars, MD

Louis Martin, MD
LSU Laparoscopic
Obesity Surgical
Specialists

George Merriman, II, MD

Surgical Specialists

Rachel Moore, MD
Surgical Specialists of
Louisiana

William Norwood, MD

John Paige, MD

William Richardson, MD
Ochsner Clinic
Foundation

Glen Steeb, MD

Michael Thomas, MD

Clark Warden, MD
Surgical Specialists of LA

Calvin Williams, MD
Advanced Surgical
Associates

Massachusetts

Limaris Barrios, MD
Beth Israel Deaconess
Medical Center

George Blackburn, MD
Beth Israel Deaconess
Medical Center

David Brams, MD
Lahey Clinic

Frederick Buckley, Jr., MD

Jonathan Critchlow, MD
Beth Israel Deaconess
Medical Center

Donald Czerniach, MD

James Ellsmere, MD
Cambridge Hospital

Burritt Haag, III, MD

James Hermenegildo, MD

Donald Hess, MD
Boston University
General Surgery

Matthew Hutter, MD
Mass General Hospital

Michael Jiser, MD

Daniel B. Jones, MD, MS
Beth Israel Deaconess
Medical Center

William Kastrinakis, MD

John Kelly, MD

David Lautz, MD
Brigham and Women's
Hospital

Edward Mun, MD
Faulkner Hospital

Dmitry Nepomnayshy, MD
Lahey Clinic

Samuel Ogle, MD

Nicole Pecquex, MD
St. Elizabeth's Medical
Center

Richard Perugini, MD
UMass Memorial
Healthcare

Kinga Powers, MD
Beth Israel Deaconess
Medical Center-Needham
Hospital

Sheldon Randall, MD

Malcolm Robinson, MD
Brigham and Women's
Hospital

Vivian Sanchez, MD
Beth Israel Deaconess
Medical Center-Needham
Hospital

Andras Sandor, MD
Commonwealth Surgical
Assoc.

Benjamin Schneider, MD
Beth Israel Deaconess
Medical Center

Roy Shen, MD
Lowell Surgical

Scott Shikora, MD
Tufts-New England
Medical Center

Rebecca Shore, MD

Michael Tarnoff, MD
New England Medical
Center

Shawn Tsuda, MD
Beth Israel Deaconess
Medical Center

Ashley Vernon, MD
Brigham & Women's
Hospital

Maryland

Andrew Averbach, MD

Scott Bovard, MD
Delmarva Bariatric Center

Brennan Carmody, MD

Joshua Felsher, MD
Inpatient Surgical
Consultants

Alejandro Gandsas, MD
Sinai Hospital of
Baltimore

Barry Greene, MD

Christina Li, MD

Peter Liao, MD

Babak Moeinolmolki, MD

Michael Schweitzer, MD
John Hopkins Bayview
Medical Center

Kuldeep Singh, MD

Michael Sofronski, MD
Delmarva Bariatric Center

Kimberley Steele, MD
Johns Hopkins

Patricia Turner, MD
University of Maryland

David Von Rueden, MD
Greater Baltimore
Medical Center

Maine

Padiath Aslam, MD

Roy Cobean, MD

Michelle Toder, MD
Northeast Surgery PA

Renee Wolff, MD

Michigan

Daniel Bacal, MD

Randal Baker, MD
Michigan Weight Loss
Specialists

Anthony Boutt, MD
Huron Surgical
Clinic, P.C.

Arthur Carlin, MD
Henry Ford Hospital

Ernest Cudjoe, MD
Great Lakes Surgical
Assoc.

Harris Dabideen, MD

Zoe Deol, MD
Michigan Bariatric
Surgery Center

Wayne English, MD
Surgical Weight Loss
Center, Marquette
General Hospital

Roche Featherstone, MD
Grand Traverse
Surgery PC

James Foote, MD
Michigan Weight Loss
Specialists

Jeff Genaw, MD
Henry Ford Hospital

Roy Hanks, DO

Steven Hendrick, MD

David Kam, MD
Bariatric Specialists of
Michigan

Paul Kemmeter, MD
Michigan Weight Loss
Specialists

Kerry Kole, DO
Real Weight Loss
Solutions, St. John
Medical Center -
Windemere Park

Kevin Krause, MD

Scott Laker, MD
Harper Hospital
Professional Building

Marek Lutrzykowski, MD

Michael Nizzi, DO
Grand Traverse
Surgery PC

Andre Nunn, MD

Farouck Obeid, MD
Hurley Medical Center

Mark Pleatman, MD

Steven Poplawski, MD

Alan Saber, MD
Michigan State University
Kalamazoo Center for
Medical Studies

Mubashir Sabir, MD

Jon Schram, MD

Michael Schuhknecht, DO
St. John Health
Riverview Center

Steven Slikkers, MD
Grand Traverse
Surgery PC

Stuart Verseman, MD
General, Vascular
Surgery and Bariatrics at
Borgess

Gary Wease, MD

John Webber, MD
Harper Univ. Hospital,
Dept. of Surgery

Michael Wood, MD

Panduranga Yenumula, MD
Michigan State University

Zubin Bhesania, MD

Minnesota

Jeffrey Baker, MD

Edmund Chute, MD
Minneapolis Bariatric
Surgeons

George Fortier, MD

Sayeed Ikramuddin, MD
University of Minnesota

Frederick Johnson, MD

Thomas Jones, MD
Park Nicollett Clinic

Todd Kellogg, MD
University of Minnesota

Michael Koeplin, MD

Howard Lederer, MD
Hennepin Bariatric Center

Daniel Margo, MD
Itasca Surgical Clinic

Walter Medlin, MD

Bradley Pierce, MD
Fairview Southdale
Weight Loss Surgery

Florencia Que, MD
Mayo Medical Center

Jeffrey Rosen, MD, MBA

Crystal Schlosser, MD
Minneapolis Bariatric
Surgeons

Michael Schwartz, MD, PhD
Minneapolis Bariatric
Surgeons

Barbara Steinbrunn, MD
Capitol Surgery PLLC

Robert Wetherille, MD
Park Nicollet Health
Services

Missouri

Roger de la Torre, MD
University of Missouri-
Columbia

Richard Follwell, DO

Ronald Gaskin, MD

Valerie Halpin, MD
Washington University

M. Hodges, MD

Lindy Hruska, MD

John Price, MD

Phillip Hornbostel, MD

Norbert Richardson, MD
Richardson Surgical LLC

J. Scott, MD
University of Missouri-
Columbia

Van Wagner, MD
Heart of America
Bariatrics

Mississippi

William Avara, III, MD
South MS Surgical
Weight Loss Center

Richard Byars, MD

Kenneth Cleveland, MD

Michael King, MD
The Center for Bariatric
Surgery

Terry Pinson, MD
Surgery Clinic of
Tupelo, P.A.

Stephen Sudderth, MD
River Region Health
System

Montana

Stephen Hennessey, MD
Great Falls Clinic, LLP

J. Pickhardt, MD

David Rohrer, MD
General, Vascular and
Laparoscopic Surgery

Charles Swannack, MD
The Montana Center for
Treatment of Obesity

Nebraska

Glen Forney, MD
Western Surgical
Group, PC

Corrigan McBride, MD
University of Nebraska
Medical Center

Dmitry Oleynikov, MD
University of Nebraska
Medical Center

Ranjan Sudan, MD

Raymond Taddeucci, MD

Thomas White, MD

Nevada

James Atkinson, MD
Surgical Weight Control
Center

Daniel Cottam, MD

Barry Fisher, MD
North Vista Hospital

John Ganser, MD
Western Bariatric
Institute

Timothy King, MD

Mark Kozar, MD
Western Surgical Group

Eugene Porreca, MD

Kent Sasse, MD
Western Surgical Group

Irwin Simon, MD

Francis Teng, MD

Robert Watson, MD

New Hampshire

Connie Campbell, MD
Catholic Medical Center

John Gens, MD
Atlantic Surgical
Associates

William Laycock, MD
Dartmouth-Hitchcock
Medical Center

Kevin Looser, MD
Portsmouth Hospital

Cynthia Paciulli, MD

New Jersey

Alexander Abkin, MD
ALSOM

Valeriu Andrei, MD
Bariatric Associates, PA

William Asihene, MD, PhD

Garth Ballantyne, MD

Frank Borao, MD

Steven Becker, MD

Nicholas Bertha, DO
Advanced Laparoscopic
Surgeons of Morris

Michael Bilof, MD

Wai Yip Chau, MD

Douglas Ewing, MD
Advanced Laparoscopic
Associates

Muhammad Feteiha, MD
Advanced Laparoscopic
Surgery of Union County

Adam Goldstein, DO

Ajay Goyal, MD

David Greenbaum, MD
Surgical Specialists of
New Jersey

Vincent Iannace, MD
Hackensack University
Medical Center

Ibrahim M. Ibrahim, MD

Richard Ing, MD

Demesvar Jean-Baptiste, MD
Bariatric Center at
Muhlenberg

Christopher Kaczmarski, MD

Wael Kouli, MD

Edward McLean, Jr., MD
Allied Surgical Group

Vishal Mehta, MD
Mehta Bariatric Center

Earl Noyan, MD

Michael Nusbaum, MD

Alexander Onopchenko, MD

Samir Patel, MD

Lyudmila Pupkova, MD
Advanced Laparoscopic
Surgeons

Ragui Sadek, MD

Hans Schmidt, MD

Jeffrey Strain, MD
Bergen Laparoscopy and
Bariatrics Associates

Karl Strom, MD

Stefanie Vaimakis, MD

Franklyn Vazquez, MD

David Ward, MD
Allied Surgical Group

Morris Washington, MD

New York

Arif Ahmad, MD
Long Island Laparoscopic
Surgery

Medhat Allam, MD

Dominick Artuso, MD
Community Hospital at
Dobbs Ferry

Marc Bessler, MD
New York Presbyterian
Hospital

Matthew Brackman, MD

Stephen Carryl, MD

Armando Castro, MD

Thomas Cerabona, MD
New York Medical
College

Edward Chin, MD

Gene Coppa, MD

John de Csepel, MD

Edward Cussatti, MD

Gregory Dakin, MD
Weill College of Medicine
of Cornell Univ.

Paul Davidson, MD
Surgical Associates of
Utica, PC

Daniel Davis, DO
Center for Obesity
Surgery

Michael Drew, MD

Michael Edye, MD

George Ferzli, MD

George Fielding, MD
NYU Medical Center

Lael Forbes, MD
University at Buffalo
Surgeons
Buffalo General Hospital

Nick Gabriel, DO
Peninsula Hospital Center
North Shore/LIJ Affiliate

Dominick Gadaleta, MD
North Shore Surgical
Specialists

Michel Gagner, MD
NY Presbyterian Hospital,
Weill College of Medicine
of Cornell University

Daniel Galvin, DO

Shawn Garber, MD

Alan Geiss, MD
North Shore Univ.
Hospital at Syosset

Larry Gellman, MD

Karen Gibbs, MD

Piotr Gorecki, MD
New York Methodist
Hospital

Kenneth Graniero, MD
Mohawk Valley

Flavia Gusmano, MD
Rochester General
Hospital

Steven Heneghan, MD
Mary Imogene Bassett
Hospital

Daniel Herron, MD
Mount Sinai School of
Medicine

Spencer Holover, MD

William Inabnet, III, MD
College of Physicians and
Surgeons of Columbia
University

Brian Jacob, MD
Laparoscopic Surgical
Center of NY

Leon Katz, MD

Ashutosh Kaul, MD
New York Medical
College

Subhash Kini, MD

John Kral, MD, PhD
SUNY Health Science
Center

Marina Kurian, MD
Manhattan Minimally
Invasive & Bariatric, P.C.

Peter Kwon, MD

Richard Lazzaro, MD

Leonard Maffucci, MD

James McGinty, MD

Heather McMullen, MD

John Mecenas, MD

Paayal Mehta, MD

Stephen Merola, MD
New York Hospital
Queens

Jeffrey Nicastro, MD

William O'Malley, MD
Highland Hospital

Joseph Patane, MD

Gary Pearlstein, MD

Alfons Pomp, MD
Cornell Weight Loss
Surgery Program

Alan Posner, MD

Colin Powers, MD
Syosset Hospital,
Laparoscopy Center

Sanjeev Rajpal, MD

Madhu Rangraj, MD

Christine Ren, MD
NYU Program for
Surgical Weight Loss

Ramon Rivera, MD
Advanced Laparoscopic
Surgical Specialists

Mitchell Roslin, MD
Lenox Hill Hospital

Aaron Roth, MD

Richard Rubenstein, MD
Caremax Surgical P.C.

P. Scalia, MD

Beth Schrope, MD
Columbia University

Paresh Shah, MD
Manhattan Minimally
Invasive and Bariatric
Surgery.

Flavia Soto, MD

Julio Teixeira, MD

Giacomo Vinces, DO

Sivamainthan
Vithiananthan, MD
Winthrop University
Hospital

Rajeev Vohra, MD

Wayne Weiss, MD
Oneonta Specialty
Services

Leslie Wise, MD
N.Y. Methodist Hospital

Jeffrey Zitsman, MD
Children's Hospital of NY
Pres.

North Carolina

Roc Bauman, MD
Carolina Weight Loss
Surgery

W. Bradshaw, MD
Regional Surgical
Specialists

Paul Carter, MD

James Classen, MD

Leland Cook, MD
Hickory Surgical
Clinic, Inc.

Monty Cox, MD
Hickory Surgical Clinic

Omar Danner, MD
Charlotte's Medical
Weight Loss Center

Eric DeMaria, MD
Duke University Medical
Center

Paul Enochs, MD
Surgical Specialists
of NC, PA

Adolfo Fernandez, Jr., MD
Wake Forest University
School of Medicine

Keith Gersin, MD
Carolinas Medical Center

Eduardo Gonzales, MD
The Surgical Weight
Loss Center

John Grant, MD
Duke University
Medical Center

Kristen Hardcastle, MD
Central Carolina Surgery

Benjamin Hoxworth, MD
Central Carolina
Surgery, PA

Timothy Kuwada, MD
Carolinas Medical Center

Kenneth MacDonald, Jr., MD
ECU, The Brody School
of Medicine

Matthew Martin, MD
Central Carolina
Surgery, PA

David Miles, MD
Miles Surgical PLLC

C. Mitchell, Jr., MD
Pinehurst Surgical Clinic

Joseph Moran, MD
Advanced Laparoscopic
Associates, P.C.

David Newman, MD

Dana Portenier, MD

Duke University

Aurora Pryor, MD
Duke Weight Loss
Surgery Center

David Voellinger, MD
Southeast Bariatrics, P.A.

Raymond Washington, MD
Pinehurst Surgical Clinic

North Dakota

Brent Bruderer, MD

Colin MacColl, MD

Timothy Monson, MD

Ohio

David Barbara, MD

Aviv Ben-Meir, MD

Stacy Brethauer, MD

Walter Cha, MD
MetroHealth Medical
Center

Bipan Chand, MD
Bariatrics & Metabolic
Institute / M61

Walter Chlysta, MD
Akron General Medical
Center

Alison Clarey, DO

Trace Curry, MD
Deaconess Surgical
Weight Loss Center

Adrian Dan, MD

Timothy Duckett, MD

Elliott Fegelman, MD
Cincinnati General
Surgeons

Victor Garcia, MD
Children's Hospital
Medical Center

Peter Hallowell, MD
University Hospital of
Cleveland

George Kerlakian, MD
Group Health Associates

Joel Korelitz, MD
Cincinnati General
Surgeons

Derrick Martin, MD
Kingsridge Medical
Center

Marc Michalsky, MD
Columbus Children's
Hospital -

Dean Mikami, MD
Ohio State University

Marcus Miller, MD
Mid-Ohio Surgical
Associates

Brian Mirza, MD

Bradley Needleman, MD
OSU Surgery, LLC

Bradley Osborne, MD
Cincinnati Weight Loss
Center

Philip Schauer, MD
Cleveland Clinic
Foundation

Kira Schofield, MD
Bariatric Wellness Center

David Schumacher, MD
Kettering Bariatrics

Mujeeb Siddiqui, DO

James Viglianco, MD

John Zografakis, MD

Oklahoma

Kevin Fisher, DO

Philip Floyd, MD

Luis Gorospe, MD

Steven Katsis, MD

Ronnie Keith, DO

JoeBob Kirk, DO

Lana Nelson, DO

Gregory Walton, MD

Oregon

Stephen Archer, MD

Clifford Deveney, MD
Oregon Health & Science
University

Mark Eaton, MD
Oregon Surgical
Specialists, PC

Neal Gorrin, MD
Oregon Bariatric Center

Dennis Hong, MD

Jay Jan, MD

Marinus Koning, MD
Advanced Surgical Care

David Maccabee, MD

Raul Mirande, MD
Southern Oregon Center
for Obesity Surgery

Robert O'Rourke, MD
Oregon Health & Science
University

Emma Patterson, MD
Oregon Weight Loss
Surgery, LLC

Salvador Ramos, DO

Steve Tersigni, MD
  Bay Bariatrics

Thomas Umbach, MD

Kenneth Welker, MD

Bruce Wolfe, MD
  Oregon Health and
  Science University,
  BTE 223

Donald Yarbrough, MD

Pennsylvania

Amjad Ali, MD

Hamot Medical Center
  Bariatric Surgery Center

Roberto Bergamaschi, MD
  Lehigh Valley Hospital

Fernando Bonanni, MD

Abington Memorial
  Hospital
  Surgical Weight Loss
  Center, Levy Plaza

Michael Bono, MD

Richard Boorse, MD
  General Surgical
  Associates, Ltd.

Alan Brader, MD
  Bariatric Specialist of PA

Anita Courcoulas, MD

Scot Currie, DO

Ramsey Dallal, MD
  Albert Einstein Medical
  Center

Luciano DiMarco, DO
  Central PA Surgical
  Assoc., Ltd.

George Eid, MD
  University of Pittsburgh

Robert Josloff, MD

Matt Kirkland, MD

James Kolenich, MD

Jeffrey Kolff, MD
  Abington Memorial
  Hospital

Christopher Kowalski, MD
  Temple University
  Hospital

James Ku, MD
  The Reading Hospital and
  Medical Center

James Luketich, MD
  Presbyterian University
  Hospital

Kim Marley, MD
  Windber Medical Center

Carol McCloskey, MD

John Meilahn, MD
  Temple University
  Medical School

Matthew Newlin, MD
  Lexington Surgical
  Associates

Victor Novak, II, MD

Pavlos Papasavas, MD
  West Penn Hospital

Anthony Petrick, MD

Robert Quinlin, MD
  Pittsburgh Bariatrics

Yannis Raftopoulos, MD, PhD
  University of Pittsburgh

Ramesh Ramanathan, MD
  Magee-Womens Hospital

Mary Reed, MD
  Geisinger Medical Center

Timothy Shope, MD
  Penn State College of
  Medicine

Paul Thodiyil, MD

Geoffrey Wilcox, MD
  Hope Bariatrics

Noel Williams, MD
  Hospital of University of
  Pennsylvania

Mark Zelkovic, MD

Rhode Island

Dieter Pohl, MD

G. Roye, MD

South Carolina

David Anderson, MD
  Advanced Surgical
  Associates

Marc Antonetti, MD
  Riverside Surgical Group

Donald Balder, MD
  Advanced Surgical
  Associates

Eric Bour, MD

Alex Espinal, MD

Edward Rapp, II, MD
  Premier Surgical
  Services, PA

Blair Rowitz, MD

Glen Strickland, MD
  SC Obesity Surgery
  Center

South Dakota

Dennis Glatt, MD

Donald Graham, MD
  Surgical Associates, Ltd.

Frederick Harris, MD
  Dakota Surgical Ltd.

Peter O'Brien, MD
  SVC - Surgical
  Associates

William Rizk, MD

Midlands Clinic

David Strand, MD
  Surgical Institute of
  South Dakota

Bradley Thaemert, MD
  Surgical Institute of
  South Dakota

Keith Vollstedt, MD
  General Surgery and
  Diagn.

Donald Wingert, MD
  Surgical Institute

Michael Wolpert, MD
  General Surgery
  and Diagn.

Tennessee

Stephen Boyce, MD
  Parkwest Comprehensive
  Weight Loss Ctr.

Mark Colquitt, MD

David Dyer, MD

Michael Hodge, MD
Surgical Group of
Johnson City, MPC

Hugh Houston, MD

George Lynch, MD

Atul Madan, MD
University of Tennessee
Health Science Center

Charles Morton, MD

Douglas Olsen, MD

Jonathan Ray, MD

Walter Rose, MD

Jack Rutledge, MD

Albert Spaw, MD

William Steely, MD

Virginia Weaver, MD
Memphis Surgery
Associates

Morris Westmoreland, MD

George Woodman, MD
MidSouth Bariatrics

Texas

Audencio Alanis, MD

John Alexander, MD

Richard Alford, MD

Richard Anderson, MD

Bruce Applebaum, MD
Southwest Surgeons for
Obesity, PA

Hugh Babineau, MD

Wade Barker, MD

Christopher Bell, MD

Richard Benavides, MD

Mary Brandt, MD

Kenneth Bryce, MD
Lone Star Lap-Band

Felipe Cantu, Jr., MD
Advanced Bariatric
Institute

Richard Carter, DO

Manuel Castro-Arreola,
MD, PhD
Southwest Surgeons for
Obesity

Ramiro Cavazos, MD
Texas Center for Medical
& Surg. Wt. Loss

Craig Chang, MD

Benjamin Clapp, MD

Stephen Clark, MD
Southwest Bariatric
Surgeons, PLLC

Richard Collier, Jr., MD

Allan Cribbins, III, MD

James Davidson, MD

Robert Davis, MD

Garth Davis, MD
Houston Surgical
Consultants

D. del Pino, MD

Patrick Dillawn, MD
Southwest Bariatric
Surgeons, PLLC

Walter Dobson, DO

Frank Duperier, MD

Steven Fass, MD
Southwest Bariatric
Surgeons, PLLC

Tim Faulkenberry, MD
Southwest Bariatric
Surgeons, PLLC

Carlos Ferrari, MD

Louis Fox, MD

Eldo Frezza, MD
Texas Tech University
Health Sciences Center

Sashidhar V. Ganta, MD

Michael Green, MD

Moya Griffin, MD

Robert Hagood, MD

Stanley Hahn, MD

David Hall, MD

Stephen Hamn, MD

Jason Harrison, MD
Texas Laparoscopic
Bariatrics, PA

Michael Helmrath, MD

Henry Horrilleno, MD
Bariatric Associates of
North Dallas

Thirumalairaj Jayakumar, MD

Nirmal Jayaseelan, MD

Jason Johnson, DO
William Beaumont Army
Medical Center

Ira Kasper, MD
QPMC, PA

David Kim, MD

Joseph Kuhn, MD

Michael Lara, MD

Philip Leggett, MD

Mario Longoria, MD

Peter Lopez, MD
University of Texas
Health Science Center

Nancy Marquez, MD
Southwest Bariatric
Surgeons, PLLC

John Marsden, MD

Robert Marvin, MD
Houston Surgical
Specialists

Marilyn Marx, MD
University of Texas
Medical Branch

John Mason, MD

Todd McCarty, MD

Robert McKinney, Jr., MD
Trinity Clinic

Fernando Miranda, MD

Adam Naaman, MD

William "Nick" Nicholson,
IV, MD

Younan Nowzaradan, MD

Paula Oliver, MD
Southwest Bariatric
Surgeons, PLLC

Nilesh Patel, MD

John Pilcher, Jr., MD

David Provost, MD
University of Texas SW
Med. Center

Paresh Rajajoshiwala, MD
Wish Center

Patrick Reardon, MD

Dana Reiss, MD

Luis Reyes, MD

Jorge Rincon, MD

David Ritter, MD

Homero Rivas, MD
UT Southwestern
Medical Center

Dirk Rodriguez, MD

Watson Roye, Jr., MD

Terry Scarborough, MD

Daniel Scott, MD
UT Southwestern
Medical Center

Michael Seger, MD

Vadim Sherman, MD

Mark Sherrod, MD
Southwest Bariatric
Surgeons, PLLC

Adam Smith, DO
Laparoscopy, Bariatrics &
Surgery, PA

Felix Spiegel, MD

Hadar Spivak, MD

Lloyd Stegemann, MD

Michel Stephan, MD

Daryl Stewart, MD

Michael Storey, MD

Jason Suits, MD
Diagnostic Clinic of
Longview

Thomas Taylor, MD
St. Joseph Medical
Center

Clifton Thomas, MD

Michael Trahan, MD
University of Texas
Medical Branch

Dexter Turnquest, MD

Frank Veninga, MD

Mark Watson, MD
UT Southwestern
Medical Center

Richard Wilkenfeld, MD

Erik Wilson, MD

Sherman Yu, MD
University of Texas
Medical School

Utah

O. Alldredge, MD

LeGrand Belnap, MD
LeGrand Belnap Surgical
Associates

Hanafy Hanafy, MD,
FRCS(Ed)

Darrin Hansen, MD

Rodrick McKinlay, MD

Christina Richards, MD

David Richards, MD
Ashley Valley Medical
Center

Steven Simper, MD

J. Speakman, MD
Southwest Surgical
Associates

Virginia

Ghiath Alshkaki, MD

Eliseo Bautista, MD
Commonwealth
Surgeons, Ltd.

Matthew Brengman, MD
St. Mary's MOB South

Thomas Clark, MD, MS

Hazem Elariny, MD, PhD
Advanced Laparoscopic &
General Surgery
Associates

Mark Fontana, MD

Troy Glembot, MD
Winchester Medical
Center Bariatric Program

Denis Halmi, MD

Paul Hogg, MD
Commonwealth Surgical
Assoc.

Andrew Kramer, DO
Appalachian Center for
Obesity Surgery

Bruce Long, MD
Carilion Surgical Care -
Brambleton

James Maher, MD
Medical College of
Virginia

Amy Martin, MD

Amir Moazzez, MD

Christopher Northup, MD
University of Virginia
Health System

Eric Pinnar, MD

Robert Sass, DO
Appalachian Center for
Obesity Surgery

Gregory Schroder, MD
St. Mary's Hospital

David Spencer, DO

Victor Stelmack, MD

Anthony Terracina, MD
Weight Loss Surgery
Center of Hampton Rds.

Daniel Tran, MD

Alan White, MD

Stephen Wohlgemuth, MD

Washington

Claudio Alperovich, MD
The Wish Center

Peter Billing, MD
Puget Sound Surgical
Center

Joseph Chebli, MD

E. Patchen Dellinger, MD
Univ. of Washington
Medical Center

Earl Fox, MD

Ki Hyun Oh, MD
St. Francis Weight Loss
Surgery Clinic

Robert Landerholm, MD
Puget Sound Surgical
Center

Ross McMahon, MD
Swedish Medical Center

Robert Michaelson, MD

Kevin Montgomery, MD

William Neal, MD
Pacific Surgical Weight
Loss Center, PLLC

Brant Oelschlager, MD
University of Washington

Myur Srikanth, MD

Lee Trotter, DO
Spokane Surgeons

Brad Watkins, MD
Northwest Weight Loss
Surgery

Andrew Wright, MD
University of Washington
Hospital

West Virginia

Charles Goldman, MD
WVU-School of Medicine

D. Nease, MD
Center for Surgical
Weight Control

Melissa Powell, MD
West VA University
Physicians of Charleston

Robert Shin, MD
Charleston Area Medical
Center Weight Loss
Center

Wisconsin

James Burhop, MD
Bariatric Institute of
Wisconsin

Manfred Chiang, MD
Bariatric Institute of
Wisconsin

Thomas Chua, MD
Wisconsin Bariatrics, SC

David Engstrand, MD
Bariatric Institute of
Wisconsin

Michael Garren, MD
UWHealth Bariatric
Surgery Clinic

Raymond Georgen, MD
Surgical Associates of
Neenah

Jon Gould, MD
UW Health Bariatric
Surgery Program

Paul Huepenbecker, MD

Matthew Johnson, MD

James Kemmerling, MD

Theresa Quinn, MD

Joseph Regan, MD

Calvin Selwyn, Jr., MD
Ministry Medical Group
Central Region

Carl Sunby, MD

Kevin Wasco, MD
Surgical Associates of
Neenah

Wyoming

Richard Fermelia, MD
Consultants in
Surgery, P.C.

M. Parnell, MD
Consultants in
Surgery P.C.

For more on Lap-Band Programs and contact information log on to
www.lapbandcompanion.com

- Web site links
- ACS accredited programs
- ASMBS accredited programs
- Available for adjustments only
- Email contacts for bariatrician and nutritionists
- Patient testimonials

Selected References

1. Angrisani L, Furbetta F, Doldi B, et al. Lap Band® adjustable gastric banding system: the Italian experience with 1863 patients operated on 6 years. *Surg Endosc.* 2003;17(3):409-412.

2. Angrisani L, Iovino P, Lorenzo M, et al. Treatment of morbid obesity and gastroesophageal reflux with hiatal hernia by Lap-Band. *Obes Surg.* 1999; 9(4): 396-398.

3. Belachew M, Belva PH, Desaive C. Long-term results of laparoscopic adjustable gastric banding for the treatment of morbid obesity. *Obes Surg.* 2002;12(4):564-568.

4. Blackburn G, Hutter MW, Harvey A, et al. Betsy Lehman Center for Patient Safety and Medical Error Reduction expert panel on weight loss surgery. *Obesity.* 2007; in press.

5. Cadiere GB, Himpens J, Hainaux, et al. Laparoscopic adjustable gastric banding. *Semin Laparosc Surg.* 2002;9:105-114.

6. Dargent J. Laparoscopic adjustable gastric banding: Lessons from the first 500 patients in a single institution. *Obes Surg.* 1999.(5):446-452.

7. *DeMaria EJ, Sugerman HJ, Meador JG, et al. High failure rate after laparoscopic adjustable silicone gastric banding for treatment of morbid obesity. *Ann Surg.* 2001;233(6):809-818.

8. Dixon JB, O'Brien PE. Health outcomes of severely obese type 2 diabetic subjects 1 1ear after laparoscopic adjustable gastric banding. *Diabetes Care.* 2002;25(2):358-363.

9. Dixon JB, Dixon AF, O'Brien PE. Improvement in insulin sensitivity and ß-cell function (HOMA) with weight loss in the severely obese. *Diabetes* 2003;20:127-134.

10. Dixon JB, Chapman L, O'Brien PE. Marked improvement in asthma after Lap-Band® surgery for morbid obesity. *Obes Surg.* 1999;9:385-389.

11. Dixon JB, Schacher LM, O'Brien PE. Sleep disturbance and obesity. *Arch Intern Med.* 2001;161:102-106.

12. Dixon JB, O'Brien PE. Gastroesophageal reflux in obesity: the Effect of Lap-Band placement. *Obes Surg.* 1999;9:527-531.

13. Dolan K, Bryant R, Fielding G. Treating diabetes in the morbidly obese by laparoscopic gastric banding. *Obes Surg.* 2003;13:439-443.

14. Edwards M, Grinbaum R, Schneider B, Walsh A, Ellsmere J, Jones DB. Benchmarking hospital outcomes for laparoscopic adjustable gastric banding. *Surg Endosc.* 2007.

15. Favretti F, Cadiere GB, Segato G, et al. Laparoscopic banding: selection and technique in 830 patients. *Obes Surg.* 2002;12:385-390.

16. Food and Drug Administration: FDA trial summary of safety and effectiveness data: The LAP-BAND® Adjustable Gastric Banding System (P000008) [article online] 2001. Available at www.fda.gov/cdrh/pdf/P000008.html. Accessed 24 August 2007.

17. Fielding GA, Rhodes M, Nathanson LK. Laparoscopic gastric banding for morbid obesity: surgical outcome in 335 cases. *Surg Endosc.* 1999;13:550-554.

18. Flegal KM, Carrol MD, Ogden CL, Johnson CL. Prevalence and trends in obesity among US adults, 1999-2000. *JAMA.* 2002;14:1723-1727.

19. Fox R, Fox K, Srikanth M, Rumbaut R. The LAP-BAND System in a North American population, *Obes Surg.* 2003;13:275-280.

20. Gastrointestinal surgery for severe obesity: National Institutes of Health Consensus Development Conference Statement. *Am J Clin Nutr.* 1992;55:S615-S619).

21. Jones DB, DeMaria E, Provost DA, et al. Optimal management of the morbidly obese patient: SAGES appropriateness conference statement. *Surg Endosc.* 2004; 18(7):1029-1037.

22. Jones DB, Nguyen N, Lopez JA, O'Brien P, Provost D. Gastric bypass and gastric adjustable-band surgery for obesity. *Contemp Surg.* 2003;59(9):403-410.

23. Jones SB, Ellenbogen J, Jones DB. Perioperative implications of obstructive sleep apnea. *Bariatric Times.* 2007:24-26, 2007.

24. Jones DB, Schneider BE. Surgical management of morbid obesity. In: Fischer JE, ed. *Mastery of Surgery.* Lippincott Williams & Wilkins; 2007:965-974.

25. Kelly J, Shikora S, Jones DB et al. Best practice updates for surgical care in weight loss surgery. *Obesity.* 2007.

26. O'Brien PE, Dixon JB, Brown W. The Laparoscopic Adjustable Gastric Band (LAP-BAND®): a prospective study of medium-term effects of weight, health and quality of life. *Obes Surg.* 2002;12(5):652-660.

27. O'Brien PE. The LAP-BAND AP System. *Bariatric Times,* 2007;4(5):24-26.

28. Ogunnaike BO, Jones SB, Jones DB, Provost D, Whitten C. Anesthetic considerations for bariatric surgery. *Anesth Analg.* 2002;95(6):1793-1805.

29. Provost DA, Ren CJ, Fielding GA, Patterson EJ, Ponce J, Smith AB, Jones DB. Laparoscopic adjustable gastric banding for morbid obesity: The US experience. *Surg Obes Relat Dis*, 2007; in press.

30. Powers K, Jones DB. *Financial impact of obesity and bariatric surgery: bariatric surgery primer for the internist*. Medical Clinics North America. 2007;91(3):321-338.

31. Ren CJ, Horgan S, Ponce J. US experience with the LAP-BAND System. *Am J Surg*. 2002;184(6B):46S-50S.

32. Ren C, Weiner M, Allen J, Favorable early results of gastric banding for morbid obesity: the American experience. *Surg Endosc*. 2004; 18(3): 543-546.

33. Sanchez V, Provost DA, DeMaria E, Blackburn G, Jones DB. Re-operative bariatric surgery. In: Callery MP (ed), *Handbook of re-operative general surgery*, Malden: Blackwell Publishing, 2006; 67-83.

34. Sarker S, Herold K, Creech S, Shayani V. Early and late complications following laparoscopic adjustable gastric banding. *Am Surg*. 2004, Feb; 70(2):146-149.

35. Schirmer B, Flum D, Schauer P, Ellsmere J, Jones DB. Bariatric training: getting your ticket punched. *J Gastrointestinal Surg*. 2007; 11:807-812.

36. Schirmer B, Jones DB. American College of Surgeons Bariatric Network: Establishing standards. *Bulletin of the ACS*; 92 (8):21-27, 2007.

37. Schneider B, Sanchez V, Jones DB. How to implant the laparoscopic adjustable band for morbid obesity. *Contemp Surg*. 2004;60(6):256-264.

38. Schneider BE, Jones DB, Provost DA. Obesity surgery: Laparoscopic Roux-en-Y and gastric band procedure. In: Jones DB, Wu J, Soper NJ (eds), *Laparoscopic surgery: Principles and procedures*, 2nd ed. New York, NY, Marcel Dekker; 2004: 553-568.

39. Shapiro K, Patel S, Abdo Z, Ferzli G. Laparoscopic adjustable gastric banding. *Surg Endosc*. 2004;18:48-50.

40. Spivak H, Anwar F, Burton S, Guerrero C, Onn A. The LAP-BAND System in the United States: one surgeon's experience with 271 patients. *Surg Endosc*. 2004;18:198-2002.

41. Wee CC, Jones DB, Davis RB, Bourland AC, Hamel MB. Understanding patient's value of weight loss and expectations for bariatric surgery. *Obes Surg*. 2006;16(4):496-501.

42. Weiner R, Blanco-Engert R, Weiner S, et al. Outcome after laparoscopic adjustable gastric banding—8 years experience. *Obes Surg*. 2003;13:427-434.

43. Vertruyen M. Experience with Lap-Band System® up to 7 years. *Obes Surg*. 2002;12:569-572.

Other Sources of Interest From Authors

1.   Jones SB, Jones DB. Patient Safety in Obesity Surgery: Defining Best Practices. Ciné-Med Publishing, Woodbury, CT, 2008.

2.   Sanchez V, Jones DB. Laparoscopic Adjustable Band. SAGES Top 14 Videos, 2nd Ed. Ciné-Med Publishing, Woodbury, CT, 2004.

3.   Jones DB, Schneider B, Blackburn G. Patient Safety in Obesity Surgery: Defining Best Practices [DVD]. Cine-Med Publishing, Woodbury, CT, 2005.

4.   Jones DB, Gagner M, Ren C, Flum D, Brunt LM. SAGES Grand Rounds: Bariatric Surgery. Cine-Med Publishing, Woodbury, CT, 2007.

5.   Jones DB, Maithel S, Schneider B. Atlas of Minimally Invasive Surgery. Cine-Med Publishing, Woodbury, CT, 2006.

Notes
on My LAP-BAND Experience

Notes
on My LAP-BAND Experience

Notes
on My LAP-BAND Experience

_____

_____

_____

_____

_____

_____

_____

_____

_____

_____

_____

_____

_____

_____

_____

_____

_____

Notes
on My LAP-BAND Experience

Index